Lifestyle Changes

12 STEP RECOVERY
NUTRITION
&
DIET GUIDE

MARILYN ROLLINS R.D.

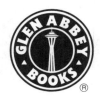

GLEN ABBEY BOOKS ®

Seattle, WA

Cover design by
    Graphiti Associates, Inc.
    Seattle, Washington

The ideas, procedures, and suggestions contained in this book are not intended as a substitute for consulting with your physician, Registered Dietitian, or qualified health care professional.

7/93

Library of Congress Cataloging-in-Publication Data

Rollins, Marilyn
        Lifestyle changes : 12 step recovery nutrition & diet guide / by Marilyn Rollins. — 1st ed.
                p.   cm.
        Includes bibliographical references.
        ISBN 0-934125-23-6 : $7.95
        1. Nutrition. 2. Twelve-step programs. I. Title.
RA784.R64   1991
613.2—dc20   91-24619
                                                                                CIP

First Edition
ISBN 0-934125-23-6
Printed in the United States of America

—————————————

10 9 8 7 6 5 4 3 2 1

DEDICATION

To all individuals and families in 12 Step
recovery who are making living amends
to themselves and others.

CONTENTS

FOREWORD

During our "addicted years," havoc has been wrought on our physical selves by our addictive behaviors. *Lifestyle Changes: 12 Step Recovery Nutrition & Diet Guide*, by Marilyn Rollins, R.D., clearly, concisely, informatively, and *sanely* outlines a means of regaining physical well-being through proper diet, exercise, rest, and diversion, not only during early recovery but also during the lifelong recovery process.

To recover from alcohol or drug dependency, eating disorders, or other "addictions" is to regain *balance* by first eliminating our chemical of choice and then, more importantly, getting in touch with our spiritual, emotional, and physical selves. Most 12 Step programs address well the regaining of the spiritual and emotional sides of our lives that need healing. The physical recovery process up until now has not adequately been emphasized by 12 Step programs or "treatment" facilities based on the A.A. philosophy.

The concepts addressed in this book should be read and embraced not only by those in recovery but also by those dedicated to helping others achieve true "sobriety," whether it be sponsors, therapists, or even those "interested" in helping one recover from his/her addiction.

SERENITY (BALANCE) =
SPIRITUAL + EMOTIONAL + PHYSICAL HEALTH

That serenity we all seek cannot be gained until *all* aspects of recovery are addressed in a balanced manner. As the Big Book says, "Are these extravagant promises? We think not. They are being fulfilled among us—sometimes quickly, sometimes slowly." There is nothing wrong with more quickly.

—George A. Streza, M.D., DABS, FACS

ACKNOWLEDGMENT AND APPRECIATION

I could not begin to thank or to mention by name or bond all my patients, friends and "adversaries," mentors, colleagues, my family-of-origin, and my "family-of-choice" who have given me their insights and presented me with so many opportunities to grow and learn. So many have taught and encouraged me as I learned about people, diets, foods, and recovery. They allowed me to have a role in, and the privilege of, sharing their lives as they struggled to overcome their personal or dietary nemeses. They have shared the celebrations of their successes and the depth of their pain as I knew them in their struggles and joys in their quest for recovery, health, balance, and serenity.

Thanks to Bill Pittman and Linda McClelland, my editors at Glen Abbey Books, for their specific help, encouragement, and professionalism.

My special gratitude and thanks to Lillian, who encouraged me personally and professionally, and always encouraged my writing; and to Chiquita, who helped me when I needed it.

My sincere appreciation, gratitude, and very special thanks to Joni, Kathie, and Judy for their love, inspiration, and encouragement, and to Bill W. for his challenges to my life.

INTRODUCTION

In 12 Step recovery we have accepted an opportunity to begin a new and improved way of life and of living. Part of this new lifestyle is improving our health and to eliminate wherever possible any effects our active addiction has had on our current and future health status. Part of improving our health, changing our life and preventing a relapse or being "stuck" in recovery is changing our nutritional status and enhancing our dietary habits.

> *"We cannot keep them from suffering; but we can keep them from suffering for the wrong reasons."* —*Anonymous*

This diet and nutrition guide is written, not for initial detoxification, but for the long-term recovery, nutrition, health, care and well-being of the individual adult. It is a framework to help prevent relapses, and to avoid some conditions that may trigger a relapse or ill health later. The basic idea is that the recovering person eat healthy, well balanced meals and snacks emphasizing complex carbohydrates, moderate protein, and reduced fat.

Bill W. (co-founder of Alcoholics Anonymous) championed appropriate nutrition in recovery; Dr. Bob (co-founder of Alcoholics Anonymous) advocated nutrition as part of the recovery process. These nutritional ideas were based on the scientific and medical knowledge, and the social patterns of the 1930s and 1940s. Although not stated as such, psychosocial and relationship issues are considered in the total recovery process and are part of the Fourth, Fifth, Eighth, Ninth, Tenth and Twelfth Step (Page 112) of many of the "anonymous" programs for addictions and recovery (Alcoholics, Al-Anon, Cocaine, Gamblers, Narcotics, Nicotine, Overeaters, Sex, etc.). Some of our psychosocial interactions and negative problems may have occurred at meal times, with food, about food or inadequacies thereof, and are corrected, over time, in similar meal time settings and interactions.

"Healthy" foods are those foods which give our bodies the nourishment, vitamins, minerals, calories, protein, fats, fiber, and fluid needed for healthy living. Unfortunately, substance abuse over time causes changes in our nutrient needs and metabolism. It also alters our nutritional needs for maintaining and enhancing our good health for the remainder of our lives.

This diet and nutrition guide is for adults. Although some of the principles advocated are suitable for children and youth who are still growing, and pregnant or nursing women in recovery, these groups have additional nutrient needs.

Substance substitution in early recovery or later may occur. This means changing the drug of choice to sugar, caffeine, nicotine, or some other substance to which you are or have become addicted. Substance substitution can maintain many of the behavioral patterns of addiction. As recovery and abstinence continue, these behavioral patterns of substance substitution need to be looked at and eliminated. This guide helps to correct and prevent substance substitution. We can't make progress in recovery by self-medicating away our problems with large quantities of ice cream, donuts, candy, or other nutritionally empty foods.

In recovery, eating disorders which were hidden by substance abuse(s) are often discovered and unmasked. The professional literature suggests that everyone in recovery be evaluated for an eating disorder, because of their susceptibility to such problems. Eating disorders include, but are not limited to, gluttony (overeating), anorexia, bulimia, and obesity.

To monitor occurrences of an eating disorder or substance substitutions, weight fluctuations, and food and meal selections are noted. Eating varied, balanced meals and snacks without sugars, excessive caffeine, or fatty foods is readily observable. Review and evaluation of a Food Diary, Record, or Journal aid in clarifying and revealing eating problems, skipping meals, excessive snacking, specific food cravings, etc.

Our "drug of choice" had different physiological and biological effects on each of us. Alcohol abuse may cause weight gain and malnutrition. Marijuana abuse may increase appetite and result in a weight gain. Heroin, morphine, and opiates alter glucose tolerance and blood sugar levels. Cocaine addiction is associated more with eating disorders, bulimia, and anorexia nervosa, and food preferences which are high in fat and caffeine. Nicotine alters the sense of taste, decreases consumption of sugars and sweets, and increases fat consumption. (In 1988, the U.S. Surgeon General specified that nicotine is an addictive substance.)

Family and social support is important in initiating and maintaining nutrition changes beneficial to improved health and relapse prevention. However, the individual is ultimately responsible for his or her own eating habits, food consumption, nutrient intake, exercise, and concomitant health status.

Our substance abuse affected our *metabolism*, which is the total of all chemical interactions that occurs in living tissue and cells. What we eat, and our *exercise and activity* level will have an effect on our health status, changes in health status, and sense of well-being. *What we eat* (time, quality, and quantity) affects our nutrient intake, changes in blood sugar, and blood chemistry.

Our attitude has a big effect on these three components. Nutrition and diet, exercise, metabolism, and attitude are very much like a pyramid: the top is your attitude and the base includes:

★ Food and liquid consumption (calories, protein, fat, carbohydrate, vitamins, minerals, fiber, and water);

★ Exercise and activity levels; and

★ Your metabolism now and as you recover and change your eating and exercise habits.

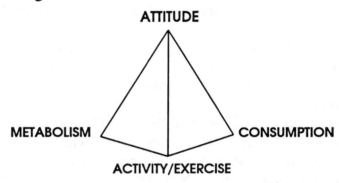

Many people have limited exercise or activity levels. Others have metabolic abnormalities which make it harder for them to eat in a spontaneous manner, and still others have excessive cravings for certain types of foods or for larger amounts of foods. These three parts—nutrition, diet, and exercise—can be balanced into changing your eating habits and patterns by altering the tip of the pyramid: **ATTITUDE**.

Our attitudes can permanently affect and improve any abnormal condition that influences our good health. It may take longer than for the "normal" person, since there are other factors which may inhibit our changes. Attitude is the overriding factor and key to our improved health, changed eating habits, and stabilization of weight at our best weight. Attitude determines whether we "walk the talk" into change and improved health, or just "talk the walk."

As with any part of your program of recovery, you can "take what you want and leave the rest." You are the one to choose which parts of any program you follow or upon which programs you embark. Your program of recovery is yours as are your nutrition and eating attitudes, beliefs, values, and habits.

EAT WELL! BE HEALTHY! BE HAPPY!

Chapter 1
DIETARY GUIDELINES

"Healthy" foods and beverages are those which give our bodies nourishment, vitamins, minerals, water, adequate calories, protein, and fats without damaging or unwholesome results. Unfortunately, substance abuse, alcoholism, eating disorders, and the continuation of these abuses for years cause changes in our nutrient needs. Good nutrition is essential to maintain or enhance good health for the remainder of our lives and the lives of our families or "significant others."

What kinds of physical, mental, emotional, or spiritual damage have the substance abuse, eating disorder, or drinking caused? What can be done to prevent further damage? What can be done to correct damage previously done? Who actually knows how to eat "appropriately"? The "isms" of alcoholism and other substance abuses are often passed from generation to generation, as are other dysfunctional family patterns, attitudes, values, habits, knowledge, and belief systems. Some people do not know healthy eating habits or food behaviors. When followed, the suggestions of this guide reduce or eliminate harmful and unhealthy effects of years of drinking and substance abuse, whether it was yours or someone else's.

Physically, because of substance abuse or poor nutritional intake, there generally has been a decrease in bone mass, changes in intestinal function, neurological (nerves) changes, elevation of total serum cholesterol, changes in cardiovascular and vascular function, alterations in blood glucose (sugar) control, and alterations in hormonal functions which affect metabolism. Some changes are reversible and can be eliminated over time. Other changes are "forever." Establishing an appropriate, healthier, and improved food program can stop or retard many of these harmful effects.

Bone mass or density does not increase in adult life. You can, through appropriate diet, stop or slow additional losses in bone density by eating adequate quantities of calcium, fluoride, and Vitamin D, and moderate amounts of protein. In women especially, bone loss in early adulthood or while bearing children can result in premature and severe osteoporosis in later years. This is one reason that 2 cups of milk (or calcium equivalents) are part of this plan. (Pregnant and nursing women require additional calcium.)

Alcohol consumption and sometimes nicotine use can cause ulcers, gastritis, malnutrition, and increased risk of cancers of the mouth, throat, esophagus, stomach, and colon. Changes in intestinal function may be reversible. This eating guide advocates reduction in or elimination of caffeine, an increase in complex carbohydrates and fiber (and therefore an increase in some vitamins and minerals), a decrease or strict limitation of the amount and kinds of fat consumed, and moderate protein intake. These suggestions, when taken, help heal the intestinal tract and its functioning.

Nicotine can play a negative and troublesome role in regulation of blood sugar. With nicotine withdrawal and abstinence, sugar cravings and binges may occur. Weight gain is not automatic for those persons who are also in recovery from nicotine addiction. Some people who quit nicotine ingestion (smoking/chewing) maintain or lose weight. To avoid weight gain after stopping nicotine, it is extremely important to eat 3 meals a day and have snacks, and eat more fruits, vegetables, and complex carbohydrates.

Changes in cardiovascular and vascular function are sometimes a function of hormonal changes, muscle wasting, or liver problems. This guide seeks to overcome these harmful effects by reducing or eliminating caffeine consumption, reducing salt intake, reducing fat and saturated fat intake, limiting sweets and sugars, and increasing fiber in the meals. Meats are either limited or eliminated to reduce the intake of saturated fat and total fats in meals.

Changes in hormonal functions caused by substance abuse sometime return to "normal" over a long time. There may be a decrease or cessation of libido. Women may have abnormal or suspended menstrual cycles. Men may have a decreased sperm count, an inability to have a "normal" erection, and an increased risk of cancer of the prostate. A "tincture of time" and a balance of protein, carbohydrate, and reduction of total fats in the diet help to reduce or eliminate these problems.

Changes in metabolism may have caused a change in blood sugar chemistry. These changes may cause a type of functional hypoglycemia or an instability of the blood sugar which can cause mood swings, minor depressive states, belligerence, hostility, rage, and inability to think in an orderly and coordinated manner ("stinkin' thinkin'"). The following nutrition and diet strategies compensate for or relieve these changes:

★ high complex carbohydrates;
★ moderate or limited amount of protein;
★ low fat and saturated fats;
★ reduction of cholesterol consumption;
★ increased fiber;
★ low "free sugars" and sweets; and
★ several snacks.

Neurological (nerves) and brain chemistry changes have affected the ability to concentrate and reason, to perceive reality, and to function harmoniously with oneself and with others. Fluctuations in blood sugar levels can also affect the ability to concentrate, to think rationally, and to be coordinated. These are other reasons to limit or eliminate sugar/

candy/sweet intake and eat three meals and two snacks each day (regardless of the work/play/meeting schedules of the individual).

Psychosocial issues of recovery which involve food, meals, and eating are rarely discussed. After completing the Fourth, Fifth, Sixth, Seventh, and Eighth Steps, Steps Nine, Ten, and Twelve can be opportunely worked at meal or snack times (after meetings) and other occasions involving food, food preparation, meals, picnics, pot lucks, eating, and restaurants.

Some of you, by the time you have read this or other parts of this book, will start your "diet babbling." "Diet babblers" are those people who discuss all about diets, possibly have tried most of them, and will argue about why "it" won't work and ignore important precepts described here. Diet babblers often "talk the walk" of diet and nutrition and do not "walk the talk." Some are professionals in the field because of their own eating disorders, substance abuse, or other dysfunctional behaviors. If you are a "diet babbler," you will want to take the easy way out and eat what you want regardless of the subsequent consequences. Perhaps you were childish, "emotionally sensitive," and grandiose and got "what you wanted when you wanted it," and food was one of those things about which you got your way. Maybe you were a "picky" or "finicky" eater and used food as a way to manipulate others or be codependent. Possibly food was a reason to use or abuse mood altering substances. Perhaps food **is** your "drug of choice" and mood altering substance, or **has become** your "drug of choice" or substitute substance in recovery.

You may have another health problem which requires special dietary measures, foods or meals; and have manipulated others because of these problems. Some of you may have a dumping syndrome, diabetes, or another health problem which requires adherence to special dietary and meal regimens as part of your health and treatment plan. For these persons, being conscientious about meals and foods is important.

However, it is not an excuse to be codependent, manipulate others, or allow others to manipulate you.

With this guide, we have the opportunity to review our eating attitudes, beliefs, and habits in great detail. We can take a "searching and fearless" inventory of ourselves and our food and nutritional attitudes and habits. We can review how this has affected others, when we were inconsiderate or self-seeking, when or where we harmed others, and when we traded "food" for favors or sex. We can be ready to have our gluttony, food, eating, or nutrition "disorders" removed.

The *Dietary Guidelines for Americans* (see Suggested Reading, p. 113) were developed by the U. S. Departments of Agriculture, and Health and Human Services. These are to guide the American public, despite significant cultural and ethnic differences, to choose and eat foods which are healthy and enhance health. Some of the nutrition and dietary guidelines, when adapted, correspond well with the objectives of recovery. The significant change from the *Guidelines* is #7: "If You Drink, Do So In Moderation"—which, for obvious reasons in recovery, is to not drink at all. Added to these are some "Just For Todays" of healthy eating habits.

★ **Eat a variety of foods:** Each day select vegetables, fruits, whole grain and enriched breads, cereals, rice, or pasta, milk, yogurt or cheese, and high protein foods, i.e., meats, poultry, fish, dried beans, or dried peas (legumes) for an adequate diet.

Since there are over 50 nutrients necessary for health and well-being, eating a variety of foods is important to get the many nutrients you require. Discussion of some of these nutrients occurs later in greater detail.

> *Just for Today: I will choose different foods I enjoy eating: vegetables, fruits, grain products, milk and milk products, high protein foods, dried beans, or dried peas.*

★ **Maintain a healthy weight:** The following chart will give you an idea about the weight range for your age. The lower weights in the range are for women; the higher weights are for men.

SUGGESTED WEIGHTS FOR ADULTS:[1]

Height	Weight in Pounds Nude (no clothes, no shoes)	
	19-34 years	35 years and over
5' 0"	97-128	108-138
5' 1"	101-132	111-143
5' 2"	104-137	115-148
5' 3"	107-141	119-152
5' 4"	111-146	122-157
5' 5"	114-150	126-162
5' 6"	118-155	130-167
5' 7"	121-160	134-172
5' 8"	125-164	138-178
5' 9"	129-169	142-183
5' 10"	132-174	146-188
5' 11"	136-179	151-194
6' 0"	140-184	155-199
6' 1"	144-189	159-205
6' 2"	148-195	164-210
6' 3"	152-200	168-216
6' 4"	156-205	173-222
6' 5"	160-211	177-228
6' 6"	164-216	182-234
6' 7"	168-221	188-239

[1]   From *Nutrition and Your Health: Dietary Guidelines for Americans.*

Your muscle mass (muscle tone), age, sex, and bone structure will influence what your "best" weight is. More detail about "best" weight and weight control is in Chapter 9.

To maintain your best health and weight, eat less fat and fatty foods, more fruits and vegetables, grains and cereals, fewer sugars and sweets, and exercise moderately 4-5 times per week.

> *Just for Today: I will set a reasonable weight goal and strive for long-term success through better habits of eating and exercise. I will seek daily progress toward my goals, not perfection.*

★ **Choose a diet low in fat, saturated fat, and cholesterol**: Select lean meats, fish, poultry, dried beans, or dried peas as protein sources. Select low-fat or skim milk products. Bake, broil or boil meats. Trim fats and skin from meats. Limit all fats, oils, and salad dressings to 3 teaspoons per day. Omit butter, sour cream, cream cheese, lard, shortening, high-fat cheeses, and fried foods. Eggs and organ meats (e.g., liver and sweetbreads) are high in cholesterol.

> *Just for Today: I will keep my cholesterol level at a desirable level with a diet low in fat, saturated fat, and cholesterol. I will follow my doctor's advice about cholesterol control. I will eat plenty of vegetables, fruits, grain products, low-fat and lean meats and dairy products, and use fats and oils sparingly.*

★ **Choose a diet with plenty of vegetables, fruits, and grain products**: Raw fruits and vegetables, whole grain breads and cereals, and dried beans and dried peas (legumes) increase dietary fiber and necessary vitamins and minerals and add variety to our meals and snacks.

Just for Today: I will eat more vegetables, dried beans and dried peas, fruits, breads, cereals, pasta, and rice. I will increase my fiber intake by eating more of a variety of foods that naturally contain fiber.

★ **Use sugars only in moderation:** Sugars include white, brown, and raw sugar, honey, syrups, and corn syrup solids. Many desserts, soft drinks, candies, and snack foods are filled with sugar. Sugary foods are proportionately higher in calories (and often fats), and are less nutrient-dense than many other sources of calories.

Just for Today: I will use sugars in moderate amounts. I will use sugars sparingly if my calorie needs are low or I need to lose weight. I will avoid excessive snacking and brush and floss my teeth regularly.

★ **Use salt and sodium only in moderation:** Salt and sodium intake may affect blood pressure. Excessive alcohol consumption may have produced high blood pressure (hypertension) which may, over time, return to normal with recovery. Recommended sodium intake for a recovering person is about 2 grams (2000 mg.) of sodium or less per day. One teaspoon of salt is roughly 2.5 grams (2500 mg.) of sodium.

Just for Today: I will maintain a healthy weight, exercise regularly, and eat less salt and sodium to maintain a healthy blood pressure. When my blood pressure is high, I will follow my doctor's advice about diet, monitoring, and medication to control it.

★ **If you are an alcoholic/addict, don't drink!** If you have abused drugs or other substances in the past, are in recovery from alcoholism, or have a family history or family members who have problems with alcohol, don't drink. If you are reading this book, you very likely fit into one or more of these categories. For those of you who are unsure about this, a review and reevaluation of your First, Fourth, Fifth, Sixth, and Tenth Steps are in order.

Sources of alcohol other than beverages and cooking wines include: some prescription and over-the-counter medications, cough syrups, decongestants, flavoring extracts, etc.

> *Just for Today: I will not use or consume any alcohol or other mood altering substance. I will eat reasonably. I will "walk the talk" of my program and be healthy and happy.*

Chapter 2
METABOLISM, CALORIES, AND CHOLESTEROL

In our days of substance abuse, we could have and probably did alter and damage our physical selves. Changes that may have occurred to our digestive system and metabolism, and the effect of and sources of calories, carbohydrates, protein, and fats are discussed below. Knowledge about what we did or could have done to ourselves is important if we are to make lifestyle changes to improve our health, nutrition, and eating program.

Digestion, Absorption, and Metabolism

Basic human anatomy is such that the intestinal tract is a series of pulverizing and extracting mechanisms. The mouth and teeth initially grind or "kibble" food into smaller particles and mix it with liquid (saliva) to be swallowed. In the stomach, acids further break the food into smaller particles and add more liquid for passage into the small intestine. The stomach is a "holding" reservoir which controls the slow release of the liquified food into the small intestine for continued segmentation and absorption into the body.

In the small intestine, enzymes from the pancreas neutralize and additionally fragment the "mushed" up food from the stomach. Absorption of amino acids, fatty acids, vitamins, and minerals occurs primarily in the intestinal tract. The lower intestines reabsorb excess fluid so wastes from the food and the intestinal mucosa (lining of the intestinal wall) are in a bulky, solid form for excretion (defecation).

Once the sub-food particles (e.g., amino acids) are absorbed into the body, metabolism takes over. "Metabolism" is the living and dying of cells. It is the action of building and rebuilding cells, parts of cells, and tissue, and the releasing and carrying away of waste and "dead" parts of cells and tissue. This process affects how much of a nutrient we need. Metabolism is the sum process of building up and breaking down cells and tissue.

Recombination of sugars, fat fragments, amino acids, amino acid chains, vitamins, and minerals into cells and nutrients for the body occurs after absorption from the intestinal tract via the blood and lymph systems. The process of digestion, absorption, and metabolism of nutrients is interwoven with the mechanical functions of the various organs through which the nutrients pass.

Damage from physical or substance (chemical) abuse to any of the organs or systems involved with the digestion, absorption, and metabolism of nutrients results in the disruption of the necessary vital functions of the body. Some of this damage may be permanent; some may be temporary.

As a result of alcoholism and substance abuse, abnormalities may occur in the mouth, esophagus, stomach, small and large intestines, liver, pancreas, heart, veins, enzyme systems, and hormonal systems which interfere with the "normal" utilization of food and nutrients. Substance abuse may have resulted in loss of or poor teeth, cancers of the mouth, esophagus or stomach, ulcers, gastrointestinal and abdominal surgeries, cirrhosis of the liver, pancreatic dysfunctions, and bowel problems.

Routine dental checks of your teeth and gums is important. Daily brushing your teeth, gums, and tongue, and flossing is suggested. Repair, replacement, or adjustments to your teeth or dentures can have a significant effect on your ability to chew and digest foods. Care of our teeth and improved dental hygiene may also be an indication of our recovery process and attitude to take better care of our total health. When you have dentures, bridges, etc., periodic adjustments or refitting may be required to assure a good fit and more comfortable chewing. Your dentist or dental hygienist can provide information regarding care of your teeth, mouth, and gums, and specific brushing and flossing techniques.

Physical examination (x-rays, blood tests, etc.) may be necessary to determine the occurrence of ulcers, reflux esophagitis, diverticulosis, diverticulitis, hernias, hemorrhoids, irritable bowel syndrome (IBS), gall bladder disease, pancreatitis or other pancreatic abnormalities, cirrhosis or other liver diseases, elevated serum cholesterol or triglyceride levels, etc. You may be constipated, or have loose or diarrheal stools. These may be the result of your substance use and abuse, poor nutrition or diet habits while using, or a particular problem that you would have had regardless of your addictive use.

Changes in nutritional status and dietary habits can alter the consequences of previous unhealthy habits. Improved diet and nutrition, balanced meals, increased fiber, and reduction of fat intake may be the key to the resolution of some of the aforementioned problems. Weight loss or gain and exercise may be another adjunct to your program of improved health.

Some health problems may not have any bearing on substance abuse. They may be a result of accidents, previous surgeries, genetics, heredity, or age. Whatever the reason, some changes in our eating and exercise habits may relieve these other health problems and change our attitude about our life, recovery, and health.

Calories, Carbohydrates, Proteins, and Fats

Carbohydrates, proteins, and fats are the origins of calories (energy) in our foods and beverages. (Alcohol is a source of calories which is now not in our plan for sobriety and health.)

There are two categories of carbohydrates: **complex** and **simple**. Proteins consist of long chains of amino acids linked together and, in foods, are commonly known as **"complete"** or **"incomplete"** proteins. Fats are sources of cholesterol, saturated, mono-unsaturated, and polyunsaturated fatty acids.

★ *Calories*

Calories are a source of fuel for us. They maintain our body heat and provide us with the energy to perform our routine activities, exercises, and normal body functions. The amount of calories we need depends on our age, sex, size (height and weight), body composition (amount of lean body mass and proportion of fat), genetic factors, energy intake, temperatures in which we live and work, and other bodily conditions.

Throughout the day, we need foods which contain carbohydrates, proteins, and fat. A good mix of daily calories is a diet of:

     55% to 70% carbohydrate;
     10% to 20% protein; and
     15% to 30% fat.

★ *Carbohydrates*

Carbohydrates are a nutrient source of calories (4 calories per gram). They are an inexpensive and easy way to obtain calories. For this healthy nutrition and diet guide, carbohydrates are 55%-70% of the total calories we eat. Complex carbohydrates are emphasized and are proportionately most of carbohydrate calories.

Complex carbohydrates are grains, pastas, breads, soy, dried beans/dried peas/lentils, and the starchy vegetables like potatoes, corn, peas, jicama, winter squashes, and yams.

Simple carbohydrates are sugars, honey, etc.

★ *Proteins*

Proteins are a nutrient source of essential amino acids and calories (4 calories per gram). Proteins are long chains of the essential and non-essential amino acids linked together. There are **nine essential amino acids.** Our bodies can make some amino acids in adequate supply for growth and regeneration of necessary body tissues. Some essential amino acids we need to eat daily so we can continue to be healthy. Too much protein may be a problem for those who have liver or kidney damage.

How big we are and our weight determines our total protein needs. We have determined our best body weight and we can readily find out what our current weight is by weighing on a bathroom scale. To estimate our total protein needs:

Multiply your best body weight by .35

Best body weight x .35 = _____

Add 10 to this number

_____ + 10 = _____ grams of total protein needed per day.

When we are more than 10% over our best body weight, then additional steps are needed to determine total protein needs. After you have completed the above calculation for your best body weight, do the same calculation using your total weight:

Multiply your current weight by .35

Current weight x .35 = _____

Find the difference between the two numbers. Divide by 2 and add this number plus 10 to equal your total daily protein needs.

[Current weight x .35] - [best weight x .35] = _____

Best weight x .35 + difference + 10 = _____ grams protein needed per day.

Extensive liver damage may require that you eat more or less protein than this basic calculation shows. This determination should be made by your physician, who has evaluated your current medical status and reevaluates it routinely, since your protein needs may shift as you maintain recovery and your liver heals.

Protein sources that contain all nine of the essential amino acids in amounts necessary for humans are **"complete"** proteins. **"Incomplete"** proteins are from those sources that do not contain all of the essential amino acids *in quantities necessary for life,* and for life and growth in children and pregnant women. Complete proteins are in foods of an animal origin. Meats, fish, fowl, dairy products, and eggs are excellent sources of complete proteins. Dried beans, dried peas (legumes), and grains are important sources of incomplete proteins. Foods that are incomplete protein sources can be combined with other foods with incomplete proteins to make the correct amino acid combination to be equivalent to a complete protein.

★ *Fats*

Fat is a nutrient source of calories (9 calories per gram) and aids in the absorption of some vitamins. "Fat" includes all fats and oils, with different chemical structures, and from different sources.

Fats are higher in calories than protein and carbohydrates and are "carriers" of the fat-soluble vitamins A, D, E and K. Fats are categorized as saturated, mono-unsaturated, and polyunsaturated. In some foods, fats are cholesterol and can have an effect on serum (blood) cholesterol levels in some people.

"Total fat" is all the fat you eat. The recommendation for total dietary fat is 30% or fewer total calories; greater restrictions (15% to 25%) may be needed to reduce elevated serum cholesterol or triglyceride levels or to reduce the risk of some cancers.

Saturated fats are those found in hardened fats such as butter and lard. The recommendation is fewer than 10% of total calories (or 4% to 6% at greater fat restrictions).

The two groups of unsaturated fats make up the remainder of the dietary fats:

Mono-unsaturated fats are fats in olive oil, peanut oil, rapeseed oil, and avocado. They are to be eaten as a greater proportion of the unsaturated fats.

Polyunsaturated fats are the fats in corn, safflower, and cotton seed oils.

Hydrogenation is a chemical process that changes liquid vegetable oils (unsaturated fat) into a more solid, saturated fat by adding hydrogen to the molecule. These fats are more stable at room temperature and so are often added to commercial products to add to storage and shelf life of the product. Not eating non-dairy creamers, fatty crackers, and chips helps to avoid this converted product and saturated fats.

Fats can affect our serum cholesterol and triglyceride levels. For healthier eating, we limit our fat and cholesterol intake. One way fats affect our arteries is in atherosclerosis. Although controversy surrounds increased longevity with a reduced fat intake, consideration of quality of life, decrease or absence of pre-menstrual syndrom (PMS), and absence of or reduction in the severity of cancers or heart disease has not been seriously and extensively studied in "at risk" populations.

Terms to become familiar with on our path of recovery and improved health are:

Atherosclerosis: A type of "hardening of the arteries" in which cholesterol, fat, and other blood components build up on arterial walls.

Lipids: Fatty substances, including cholesterol and triglycerides, that are present in blood and body tissues.

Triglycerides: These are the major kind of fat in foods. These fats add texture to foods, and aid in the absorption of fat-soluble vitamins. Serum triglycerides are a part of the fats in the blood and, in heavy drinkers and practicing alcoholics, may be significantly elevated. In sobriety, these serum triglyceride levels may return to normal.

Lipoprotein: Protein-coated packages that carry fat and cholesterol through the blood. Lipoproteins are classified according to their density.

High density lipoprotein (HDL): also known as "good" cholesterol, helps to eliminate cholesterol from the blood stream. The higher your HDL level is the better it is. Women, as a result of "female" hormones, generally have higher HDL levels than men.

Low density lipoprotein (LDL): also known as "bad" cholesterol, forms plaque in the arteries and is the cause of atherosclerosis.

Cholesterol

Cholesterol is a soft, waxy substance found in some foods. It is manufactured in the liver, and is necessary for the production of hormones, bile acid, and Vitamin D. Liver damage may affect the amount of cholesterol made.

Blood (serum) cholesterol: recommended levels are less than the upper limit of normal on the specific test equipment print-out, or fewer than 200 mg/dl, whichever is lower.

Dietary cholesterol: When serum cholesterol is elevated, initially a reduction to fewer than 300 mg/day cholesterol and reduction of fat is advised. Additional restrictions may be recommended to reduce cholesterol consumption to 100 to 150 mg/day and restrict total fat to less than 20%/day.

Omega-3 fatty acids are a very special type of fatty acid found predominantly in cold-water, deep-sea fish such as mackerel. Omega-3 fatty acids are readily obtained by having fish at a meal at least four times a week as your source of high protein food.

When there has been liver damage from substance abuse or any other reason, there often is an elevation in serum cholesterol which requires a diet lower in cholesterol. Eggs, liver, other organ meats, and cheeses are diligently avoided.

In a varied and balanced diet program, your meals and snacks include carbohydrate, protein, and fat. The Five Food Clusters of Dried Beans/Dried Peas/Lentils, Milk, Fruits and Vegetables, Breads, Grains and Cereals, and High Protein incorporate these ideas for your ready implementation and ease of understanding. (These are explained in detail in Chapter 5.)

Chapter 3
VITAMINS AND MINERALS

Vitamins and minerals are essential nutrients for vital functions in your body. They may be part of a cell (red blood cells, protein tissues, immune system, hormones, etc.) or essential for biochemical reactions (metabolism). Vitamins are "vital" for life. They are the "helpers" that aid in digestion, absorption, and metabolism, and sometimes are built into body structures.

The specific reactions of vitamins help us function and maintain our normal body temperature and energy levels. Vitamin B deficiencies produce symptoms in the **gastrointestinal tract** (diarrhea, nausea, vomiting, anorexia, and stomach upset); **nervous system** (mental confusion, irritability, insomnia, fatigue, depression, and muscle pains); **muscles** (wasting, weakness, and muscle pain); **cardiovascular system** (enlarged heart, abnormal heart action, and edema); **skin and mouth** (dermatitis, cracks at the corners of your mouth, irritation of sweat glands, loss of hair, dryness, and redness, smoothness and swelling of the tongue); and **eyes** (redness and hypersensitivity to light).

Many of us had these symptoms during our months or years of substance abuse. They may have been directly attributed to our poor nutrient intake during that time, or as a direct result of the changes in metabolism that occurred because of our drug of choice. As our body heals, and we get past the first thirty days of recovery, these symptoms may reverse and be totally eliminated with our change in attitude, and a balanced and varied diet.

Minerals are generally part of various cells and part of the functioning of that particular cell. Calcium and iron are two very necessary and vital minerals which are frequently not eaten in adequate quantities for the best of health.

It is necessary to consume vitamins and minerals on a routine basis. There are fat-soluble and water-soluble vitamins, major minerals, and trace elements.

Vitamins

Fat-soluble vitamins (A, D, E, and K) are generally eaten in more than adequate amounts by persons who eat a variety of vegetables, fruits, fish, and milk. Some fats and oils contain fat-soluble vitamins. Excessive storage of fat-soluble vitamins and overdoses can occur, especially with vitamin supplementation. These vitamins can accumulate over years to reach toxic levels.

Vitamin A is necessary in visual adaptation to light and dark and in resisting infections. It is available in *dark green and deep yellow or orange vegetables, and in orange and some red fruits.* Vitamin A is measured in retinol equivalents (RE), and includes betacarotene, a "precursor" or provitamin of Vitamin A.

The absorption and utilization of calcium in the maintenance of bone integrity requires **Vitamin D**, which is made from serum cholesterol in sunlight. In parts of the country where you are outdoors in the sunshine, there is adequate conversion of cholesterol to Vitamin D without requiring significant amounts in your diet. *Milk and milk products* are often fortified with Vitamin D.

The functioning of cells requires **Vitamin E**. Vitamin E is measured in Tocopherol Equivalents. Deficiencies of Vitamin E can cause neurologic abnormalities and reproductive problems. Vitamin E is found in *vegetable oils and green, leafy vegetables.*

Vitamin K is necessary for normal clotting of blood. Adequate Vitamin K intake is very important in individuals who take anticoagulants (e.g., in the treatment of heart disease), or who may be consuming excessive amounts of Vitamin E. Vitamin K is found in *green, leafy vegetables, milk, meats, eggs, cereals, and fruits.* It is made in the intestinal tract by the normal flora.

Water-soluble vitamins are Vitamin C, and the "B" complex vitamins of thiamine, riboflavin, niacin, pantothenic acid, pyridoxine (B_6), folacin, B_{12} (cyanocobalamin), and biotin. Niacin is measured in Niacin Equivalents and is sometimes used in pharmacological (medicinal) doses to reduce serum cholesterol levels. Water-soluble vitamins are in a variety of vegetables, fruits, enriched or whole grains and cereals, and some meats.

Vitamin C or ascorbic acid is needed to maintain the functioning of connective tissue and blood vessels, healing of wounds, normal protein metabolism, and to combat stress. Vitamin C aids in the absorption of iron in the intestinal tract and is essential for the metabolism of several amino acids and iron, including promotion of the development of the matrix of teeth and bones. Vitamin C is commonly known for its prevention of scurvy. Megadoses of Vitamin C (which can occur when taking vitamin supplements) is thought to result in the formation of kidney stones, abdominal cramps, or nausea, and may interfere with or destroy several other vitamins (B_{12} and E).

Fresh, rapidly growing fruits and vegetables are high in Vitamin C. These include broccoli, Brussels sprouts, collards, guava, horseradish, kale, turnip greens, sweet peppers, and potatoes. Fruits high in Vitamin C include citrus (oranges, grapefruit, etc.), acerola cherries, cantaloupe, and strawberries.

Thiamine, niacin, riboflavin, pantothenic acid, B_6, and B_{12} are necessary in protein and energy metabolism. Folacin, B_6, and B_{12} are essential for the production of red blood cells. (Deficiencies of these three vitamins can result in anemia.) Energy expenditure determines the physiological requirements of thiamine, niacin, and riboflavin since these vitamins are a necessary part of energy metabolism. With increased energy expenditure and exercise, calorie and food needs increase, so consuming additional complex carbohydrates in the form of whole grain or enriched breads and cereals more than compensates for the increased nutrient needs.

Folacin and B_{12} regenerate new tissue and replenish tissue in the gastrointestinal tract. (Deficiencies of these two vitamins can result in deterioration of the GI tract.)

Also, Vitamin B deficiencies produce abnormal symptoms in the gastrointestinal tract, nervous and cardiovascular systems, muscles, skin, tongue, mouth, and eyes.

Thiamine is in *enriched or whole grain breads, cereals, pastas, dried beans and dried peas, milk, and pork. Milk and meat* are the main sources of **riboflavin**. **Niacin** is in *milk, eggs, meat, poultry, fish, and enriched or whole grain breads and cereals.* **Vitamin B_6** is in *meats, legumes, vegetables, some fruits, and whole grain cereals.* **Folacin** is in *legumes, some fruits and vegetables* including asparagus, broccoli, Brussels sprouts, corn, green peas, orange juice, and winter squash. **Vitamin B_{12}** is in *fermented soy products* and "animal" products, i.e., *meats, milk, cheeses, and eggs.* Since the B Vitamins of **pantothenic acid** and **biotin** are so widely distributed in foods, eating a varied diet provides an adequate amount of these two vitamins.

Supplementation with water-soluble vitamins is unnecessary on a daily basis. Despite the fact that these are water-soluble and excesses are excreted in your urine, there normally is an adequate "floating" supply of these vitamins in the body when we eat a well-balanced diet from the basic five Food Clusters.

Minerals

Minerals include major minerals and trace or micronutrient elements. The action of minerals is dependent on the availability and amount of other minerals and nutrients either in your body or in the foods you eat. With excessive magnesium, calcium is less readily absorbed and retained, Vitamin C enhances iron absorption, and excess zinc decreases the utilization of copper.

Major minerals are: calcium, phosphorus, magnesium.

Trace or micronutrient elements are: iron, iodine, selenium and zinc. Other possible micronutrient elements are aluminum, antimony, arsenic, barium, boron, bromine, cadmium, chromium, cobalt, copper, gallium, lead, lithium, manganese, mercury, molybdenum, nickel, rubidium, silicon, silver, strontium, tin, titanium, and vanadium.

Eating a variety of foods each day from the five Food Clusters provides an adequate amount of these minerals in an appropriate balance for absorption, utilization, healing, health, and recovery.

Calcium is a part of bone development and maintenance, and muscle and blood formation. It has a role in transmission of nerve impulses, maintenance and function of cell membranes, and activation of enzyme reactions and hormone secretion. It appears to have a role in maintaining normal blood pressure and explicitly contributes to bone density and strength.

Approximately 99% of the body's calcium is in the bones. Despite common belief, bone mass is constantly undergoing change and turnover. Bone mass begins to deteriorate in our forties and fifties. This deterioration continues into older age, and can cause crippling bone deformities and irreparable fractures. Utilization of calcium depends also on protein intake, Vitamin D, extent of sunlight exposure, Vitamin A, phosphorus intake, fiber content of your diet, and daily intake of fluoride and minerals other than calcium. Eating large amounts of protein foods causes increased losses of calcium instead of its continued reabsorption and utilization.

Milk and milk products are a major source of calcium. When you do not choose milk or milk equivalents, you need to emphasize other foods that have a significant calcium content; i.e., canned salmon or sardines with bones, dark leafy green vegetables, broccoli, bok choy, and tofu.

Phosphorus is part of bones, blood, and cells, and is required for effective use of many of the B vitamins and in energy metabolism. Phosphorus is in *almost all foods*. Excessive and prolonged use of nonabsorbable antacids causes a phosphorus deficiency which results in weakness, bone pain, anorexia, and lassitude. (Self-medicating of ulcers or other "stomach" problems can be hazardous and damaging to your health and recovery.)

Magnesium is needed in protein metabolism, energy production, and your enzyme system, and also helps prevent tooth decay. Magnesium is in *cereal grains, dark green vegetables, seafood, and dried beans and peas.* Magnesium deficiency is thought to cause the hallucinations that occur in withdrawal from alcohol.

Iron carries oxygen to the cells, bones, and muscles, and is part of many enzymes. Since most of the iron is in blood, losses of blood via ulcers, wounds, or menstruation can cause iron deficiency.

The practicing alcoholic may have an excessive amount of iron since alcohol consumption increases iron absorption from the intestinal tract. Ingestion of potentially harmful amounts of iron occurs when vitamin/mineral "supplements with iron" are taken in the mistaken belief that they will counterbalance any "malnourishment" caused by substance abuse or poor eating habits or both. Tissue damage, especially to the liver, occurs as a result of excessive iron absorption (and substance abuse). The risk of infections increases because of the iron-rich blood supply and the body's weakened defense system.

Meats, fish, poultry, dried beans and dried peas, whole grain, enriched and fortified grains and cereals, dark green leafy vegetables, and dried fruits are high in iron. Cooking with an iron skillet (uncoated, unenameled) adds to the iron available for absorption. Simultaneously eating Vitamin C-rich foods aids in the absorption of iron. Eating a variety of foods also assures an adequate iron intake. *Liver, organ meats, and eggs* are high in iron (and also high in cholesterol).

An iron supplement is often recommended for women who can bear children or are pregnant. This ought to be discussed with your physician since excessive iron consumption causes constipation, and potentially, continued harm to an already damaged liver.

Zinc is necessary for the normal metabolism of carbohydrates, protein, and fat, the production of cells and sperm, healing and immune reactions, growth and maturation in children, smell, taste, and sensitivity to flavors in foods. Foods high in zinc are *meats, shellfish (especially oysters), dried beans and dried peas. Whole grain breads and cereals and milk* contain some zinc and will add to zinc to your diet when eaten in sufficient quantities. *Liver* is high in zinc (and also high in cholesterol).

Iodine is necessary for synthesis of the thyroid hormones. Thyroid hormones regulate body temperature, metabolism, use of oxygen, and functioning of nerves and muscles. *Seafood* is an excellent source of iodine. Use of *iodized salt* is an important supplement to avoid deficiency. Low thyroid output can be a cause of lethargy and weight gain. If this is a concern to you, ask your physician to complete the appropriate tests to determine your thyroid hormone status. It is well known that thyroid deficiencies are rarely responsible for overweight. Overeating and under-exercising are the common culprits of excess weight.

Sodium is important in fluid maintenance in your body. *Salt* is the most common form of sodium. Cured (e.g., ham), pre-prepared (e.g., canned or frozen dinners), pickled (e.g., sauerkraut), or highly seasoned (e.g., oriental and Mexican) foods usually contain most or all the sodium that you require for that day.

Sodium may be harmful in excessive quantities. In some people, excessive consumption of sodium and table salt can contribute to high blood pressure (hypertension). Often high blood pressure is better controlled when you reduce your total intake of salt and sodium from all sources. For the very careful, check the local water supply to determine the sodium content in your water supply at home and work. Sodium may also be added to your water via a water softener system.

Selenium is required in some specific metabolic reactions. There is some evidence that a low selenium intake for a long time can produce some kinds of heart abnormalities. There are also case reports of the toxic effects of high intakes of selenium which result in nausea, changes in nails, irritability, and fatigue.

Seafood is an excellent source of selenium. *Some meats and grain* are good sources of selenium. The amount of selenium in grains, fruits, and vegetables depends on the selenium in the soil.

The trace elements of **aluminum, antimony, arsenic, barium, boron, bromine, cadmium, chromium, cobalt, copper, gallium, lead, lithium, manganese, mercury, molybdenum, nickel, rubidium, selenium, silicon, silver, strontium, tin, titanium,** and **vanadium** interact in metabolism and are distributed in a variety of foods.

To obtain a balance of all the nutrients (more than 50 of them), eat, in moderation, a variety of dried beans and dried peas, fruits, vegetables, breads, grains and cereals, meat, fish, and poultry, and drink milk.

Vitamins and minerals, when taken in large enough doses, can produce toxic and pharmacological (medicinal) reactions. Pharmacologic function of a very high dose of vitamin is usually not the same as the nutrient or physiological function. Some vitamins or minerals may be recommended to you by your physician to treat a specific medical problem. However, even in these cases, there is the potential for toxic and detrimental side effects, especially when taken for a long period of time. (See Chapter 4.)

Chapter 4
FIBER, ADDITIVES, CAFFEINE, SUPPLEMENTS, AND SWEETS/SUGARS

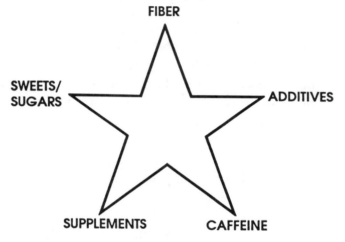

We now start to review some of the specific guidelines to healthier eating in recovery, to help eliminate a relapse, and for longevity. We begin with fiber, additives, caffeine, supplements, and sweets and sugars. Other topics which can help our lifestyles to better health include foods, meals, shopping, emotional needs, and exercise.

Fiber

Fiber is a "nutrient" that we ought to be consuming routinely. Fiber is necessary to maintain or increase intestinal motility (movement) and to produce normal bowel habits. It reduces the risks of certain cancers and heart diseases. Fiber helps to:

★ retain water in the intestinal tract to relieve constipation;

★ prevent increased abdominal pressure and enlarged veins;

★ prevent straining on defecation which may lead to hemorrhoids;

★ exercise the muscles of the digestive tract to retain health and muscle tone, and withstand internal bulging (diverticulosis);

★ speed the passage of food and waste materials through the digestive tract to reduce the time of tissue exposure to possible cancer-causing agents in the foods;

★ bind bile salts in the intestinal tract for excretion;

★ bind fats and cholesterol to help reduce blood cholesterol and triglycerides levels and possible risk of heart and artery disease;

★ regulate blood sugar control by reducing sharp increases of blood sugar and by reducing insulin needs; and

★ lose weight.

Fiber is categorized as either **soluble** or **insoluble**. Soluble fibers are cellulose, hemicellulose, and lignin; insoluble fibers are gums, mucilages, and pectin. These fibers are in fruits, vegetables, dried beans and dried peas, grains, and meats. Eating a variety of these foods each day provides a suitable balance of the kinds of fiber necessary. Eating fresh and raw vegetables and fruits, and whole *grain* breads and cereals increases our intake of fiber. The fiber in apples, blackberries, and oat bran helps to reduce cholesterol. The fiber in whole grains and cereals, some vegetables and fruits, dried beans, and dried peas increases intestinal activity and helps maintain the muscles in the intestinal walls.

Along with fiber, it is necessary to have an adequate intake of **water** and **fluids**. Drinking sufficient water eliminates waste products from your blood stream, intestinal tract, and lungs. It also aids in cooling your body to maintain normal body temperature. Drinking 8 to 12 glasses or more of water a day is adequate. Water helps prevent fluid retention, replaces fluids lost during exercise, and eliminates potential problems of dehydration.

Additives

Food additives are useful in maintaining a safe and adequate food supply. Many foods have additives that help maintain the shelf life of the product or enhance our eating enjoyment by smell, taste, or appearance. Several of the very common (and centuries-old) additives/preservatives are salt, sugar, and vinegar. (Vinegar is the preservative in sauerkraut and kim chee, a Southeast Asian cabbage.)

Commercially prepared foods commonly have seasonings (herbs, spices), flavoring extracts, food dyes or whiteners, and stabilizers (e.g., hydrolyzed vegetable protein) added to them besides salt, sugar, or vinegar. Oils in foods are sometimes "hydrogenated" to retard spoilage and extend the shelf life of the product. Additives are also in such common foods as bread and cereals.

Knowing what we're eating helps us make healthier food choices. Reading the list of ingredients on labels of packaged foods gives us an idea of the number and extent of additives. We can make an informed decision about what we eat and what effect it will have on us, our health (blood pressure, cholesterol, weight, etc.), or our recovery process.

Salt is a preservative and flavoring agent. Some foods which have a high salt (sodium) content include: monosodium glutamate (MSG); barbecue, soy, steak, teriyaki, and Worchestershire sauces; dehydrated gravy, sauce and soup mixes; pickles; other relishes; clear broth, bouillon, and consommes; and canned or dehydrated soups (e.g., chicken noodle, vegetarian, etc.).

Foods high in salt and fat include: canned cream soups, chowders, soups with ham, olives, most frozen "TV" dinners, Hollandaise sauce, cream and cheese sauces, taco and enchilada sauces, potato, corn, and snack chips, and mixes like taco mix, Hamburger Helper®, macaroni and cheese, etc.

Caffeine

Apply the "rule of three": no more than 3 servings of caffeinated foods/beverages per day. Another recovery health habit to follow is to avoid caffeine after 2:00 pm, or within 8 hours of your normal time to go to sleep. Some physicians feel that consuming more than 250-300 mg. caffeine per day is a pharmacological or drug dose of caffeine which produces strong stimulating effects. Be careful that you are not using caffeine or coffee as a substitute substance in your recovery.

Coffee has about 115 mgs. of caffeine per eight-ounce cup. Heavy use of caffeine (more than 8-10 cups of coffee or glasses of iced tea per day) can cause anxiety, hyperactivity, dizziness, insomnia, headache, jitters, tremors, and irritability. Other side effects of caffeine include increased heart rates and metabolism, changes in the elasticity of arteries, relaxation of autonomic muscles (respiration, intestinal tract, and kidneys), stimulated production of gastric secretions, and increased hunger or feelings of the need to eat to excess more often. High caffeine consumption is thought to contribute to osteoporosis. Caffeine stimulates a release of insulin which can cause hunger more quickly and stimulate the deposit of fat tissue.

It is recommended that people with chronic fatigue syndrome and women with PMS or fibrocystic breast disease avoid caffeine entirely.

There are times in our recovery and during periods of significant stress and tension that problems of sleeping or relaxing occur. Caffeine consumption may contribute to our poor sleep or rest habits. Often at meetings (and especially night meetings), coffee is the only beverage available. Better choices for beverages at meetings are water and decaffeinated coffee.

Caffeine-containing foods/beverages are coffee, teas, some herbal teas (e.g., Celestial Seasonings), diet or regular colas, chocolates (milks, candies, bittersweet, and baking), cocoa, cacao, guarana (Brazilian), mate (Argentinean), or foods that contain any of these items. Some over-the-counter drugs contain caffeine and should be excluded or counted as part of our daily caffeine consumption. Drugs with caffeine include **pain relievers** (e.g., Anacin, Empirin); **allergy or cold remedies** (e.g., Dristan); **stimulants** (e.g., No Doz); and some **"diet" pills.**

Caffeine is a stimulant and can have a significant effect on us whether we realize it or not. Excessive consumption of caffeine may result in increased hunger and feeling a need to eat more food, more often. Some persons are particularly sensitive to any caffeine and start "bouncing off walls" when they have even **one** caffeine-containing beverage or food. For these persons, complete abstinence from all caffeine is a wise and prudent choice.

Decaffeinated beverages and herbal teas may contain other stimulants or chemicals (such as theobromines and theophylline) that will have an adverse effect on you. They may affect your new nutrition program when consumed in large quantities or strong, well steeped mixtures. Herbal teas may cause diarrhea, contribute to high blood pressure, or be known carcinogens and toxins. Components that affect the chemical content of herbal teas and their effect on us include: the age of the leaves when picked; if leaves, branches, or bark are in the "tea"; storage time and conditions before steeping; how long the tea is steeped; how much we drink; and how rapidly we drink it.

Postum (a non-caffeine, cereal beverage), when consumed in large quantities, may cause gas or act as a laxative.

Supplements

Vitamin, mineral, and protein or amino acid supplements
are unnecessary after detoxification (and are not necessarily
needed during detoxification). Your physician can make the
best recommendation as to supplements. Some minerals may
have accumulated in excessive amounts because of abnormal
liver metabolism during alcohol or substance abuse.

Excessive protein intake or extra amounts of these minerals in the form of supplements are harmful and can cause
additional liver damage. "Protein pills" often contain 0.5
grams or less of protein, and 14 to 20 tablets are required to
yield the amount of protein contained in 1 ounce of meat or 1
cup of milk.

Excessive consumption of certain vitamins may cause or
intensify particular gastrointestinal problems. Excessive Vitamin A intake over years can cause irreversible bone deformities. Excessive Vitamin D can cause additional liver
damage.

Persons in recovery and those with obsessive, compulsive,
or addictive personality characteristics often become obses-
sive-compulsive-addictive about nutrient intake and supplementation. We can accept our body as it is, change the food we
eat and have available, and exercise to positively affect our
recovery, health, and metabolic status.

In reality, you may be saying that you *need* a vitamin
supplement and you are going to find one or more and take
them. When you are eating a balanced, varied diet, supplementation could easily be excessive. Therefore, my caution is: if
you insist and plan to take a supplement:

> ★ select one with the greatest variety of vitamins and
> minerals;

★ with none of these vitamins and minerals in excess of 100% of the U. S. RDAs;

★ take them no more often than twice per week; and

★ purchase them at a general drug or grocery store (not a health food store, because of cost and claims made about products which may not be true).

This will provide you with the protection you *think* you need, and help to reduce or prevent any potential damage extra nutrients may cause. Read the labels of the brand names and house brands, and compare them with each other for vitamin and mineral variety and amount, and cost per pill or capsule.

Claims made about a supplement which are *not* on the label are often misleading or untrue. There are strict regulations about information that can be put on a label. Claims on a label are substantiated by accepted research methods. Claims *not on the label* could include commercial "hype" to sell the product at a frequently blown up price.

Sweets/Sugars

These can replace essential nutrients. Some sugar substitutes may cause metabolic changes in the brain which could result in "stinkin' thinkin'" and relapse. Sugary foods when eaten alone may cause unwanted, unsuspected, and "abnormal" shifts in our blood sugar (and therefore in our attitude and mood).

There is postulation that sugars and sweets increase the cravings for some, if not all, of the drugs-of-choice that we abused. For instance, sweets can increase the craving for cocaine in those recovering from cocaine abuse. In this context, avoiding sweets and sugars then can become a very significant factor in our continued program of recovery.

Recent research suggests that sugars and sweets adversely affect women with PMS. Reduction or elimination of sugar throughout the month may reduce the "craziness" associated with PMS and therefore the emotional upheaval, distress, and potential desire to return to previous substance abuse patterns or practices.

Although sugar substitutes do not add many calories, each time they are consumed the taste for sweets is reinforced. This reinforcement occurs regardless of the source of the item, whether it be diet sodas or "diet" candies. The more sweet flavor we eat, the more we want to eat and the more we emotionally desire.

Sugars and ingredients which are sugars include: brown sugar, confectioner's sugar, corn sweeteners, corn syrup, high-fructose corn syrup, dextrose, fructose, galactose, glucose, sucrose (granulated sugar or table sugar), honey, invert sugar, lactose, levulose, maltitol, mannitol, sorbitol, xylitol, maltose, maltodexterines, maple sugar, molasses, natural sweeteners, raw sugar, and turbinado sugar.

Other foods which contain large amounts of sugar are jellies, jams, marmalades, preserves, honey, molasses, syrup, pure sugar candies such as hard candy, gum drops, jelly beans, marshmallows, and plain mints.

Making selections of some foods which have sugar(s) listed after the first four ingredients is acceptable. By reading labels, we can make this healthy decision since sugar will not be a significant ingredient in that product.

There are now several sugar substitutes on the market, with the prospect of more to be approved by the Federal Drug Administration (FDA) soon. FDA approval for these items includes in which products or types of products they may be used. Other countries allow some sugar substitutes not approved for use in the United States. Sugar substitutes are saccharin, aspartame (Nutrasweet), and acesulfame K.

When we are adhering to a reduced fat and or lower cholesterol diet plan, the following information is helpful.

Fat-free and low-fat desserts and sweets include: Angel food cake, gelatin desserts, sherbet (1-2% fat), fruit and Italian ice, sorbet, popsicles, fat-free frozen yogurt, pudding made with skim milk, chocolate desserts made with cocoa powder and without eggs or other sources of fat, meringue, fat-free gelatin mousse, and those without nuts, sauces, or cream. Licorice, although low in fat, is known to raise blood pressure when eaten in large quantities.

High-fat desserts and sweets include: Commercial or conventional cakes, pies, cookies, ice cream, ice milk, frozen tofu; any dessert containing cream, shortening, coconut, or saturated fats; butter-cream or whipped cream frostings; frozen desserts made with saturated fats; chocolate desserts or those with cocoa butter; any with nuts; bombe; parfait; mousse; chocolate candies; candy bars; milk chocolates, bittersweet, dark and white chocolates; hot cocoa mixes; Ovaltine®.

POINTS TO REMEMBER

★ Foods high in fiber are dried beans, dried peas, lentils, whole grain breads and cereals, and some raw fruits and vegetables.

★ Additives to foods retard spoilage, but can be harmful to some people.

★ Limit caffeine to no more than 3 caffeine-containing foods/beverages per day.

★ Eat a variety of foods which contain the vitamins, minerals, protein, fiber, and other nutrients necessary.

★ Replace sweets and sugars with additional fruits, vegetables, breads, cereals, and grain products to improve nutrient intake.

Chapter 5
FOOD CLUSTERS—THE BASIC FIVE

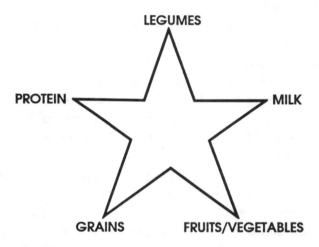

LEGUMES

PROTEIN

MILK

GRAINS

FRUITS/VEGETABLES

The basic Food Clusters provide a balance of nutrient-dense, foundation foods in an easy, simple way. The Clusters include Dried Beans/Dried Peas/Lentils (Legumes), Milks, Fruits and Vegetables, Breads, Grains and Cereals, and High Protein foods. Additional foods are often eaten which add fats, calories, and possibly other ingredients which can be harmful to your general good health, longevity, and sense of well-being.

Dried Beans/Dried Peas/Lentils (Legumes)

★ *Servings per day: At least one 1/2 cup portion.*
Select additional amounts from this Cluster when you desire more calories, complex carbohydrates, or fiber. Also,

if you decide to be a lacto-ovo-vegetarian (not eating flesh of animals or fish), substitutes for the "Meat/High Protein" Cluster are in this Cluster.

Dried beans, dried peas, and lentils are also known as legumes or pulses. The low-fat items in this Cluster include baked beans, black beans (turtle beans), garbanzo (chick peas), kidney, lima, pinto or calico, black, navy, red, white, pink beans, black-eyed (cow) peas or lentils, split peas, and soybeans and tofu (soybean curd).

Dried beans/dried peas/lentils are not only high in complex carbohydrates but also a good source of fiber, protein, calcium, and iron.

Ways to incorporate beans into the meals are: soups (i.e., lentil, split pea or navy bean), stews, casseroles, kidney or garbanzo bean salads, stir-fry items, chili con carne, ranch-style beans, and lima beans, or pureed for spreads or dips. Some international dishes which contain dried beans/dried peas/lentils as a main ingredient are minestrone soup, Boston baked beans, Senate Navy Bean soup, miso, humus (humous), dal, refried beans, chili with beans, and pasta é fagiole.

It is advisable to eliminate the very high-fat foods in this Cluster: nuts (almonds, Brazil, cashews, coconut, filberts, peanuts, pecans, pignolia [pine nuts], walnuts), and seeds (pumpkin, sesame, and sunflower).

Milk

This Cluster includes skim milk, low-fat milks (1% and 2%), and plain low-fat yogurt.

★ *Servings per day: two 1-cup portions or calcium equivalents.*

Milk products are important sources of calcium and protein. They add riboflavin, zinc, and folacin to your meals. Fortified milk is a significant source of Vitamin D.

Cheeses substitute for milk to obtain the nutrients of calcium, protein, zinc, and riboflavin. Cheeses have relatively less calcium than milk with varying amounts of fats, saturated fat, and cholesterol. The cheeses lowest in fat are: cottage cheese, grated Parmesan cheese, diet cheeses (low-fat cheeses with fewer than 55 calories per ounce), and pot cheese. Skim or part-skim milk cheeses such as ricotta, mozzarella, and diet cheeses (56 to 80 calories per ounce) are higher in fat.

The cheeses highest in fat are "regular" cheeses, such as American, Bal Paese, Blue (Bleu), Boursault, Brick, Brie, Camembert, Caraway, Caciocavallo, Cheddar, Colby, Dolfino, Edam, Feta, Fontina, Formage de chevre, Gjetost, Gorgonzola, Gouda, Greyerzer, Gruyere, Liederkranz, Liptauer, Limburger, Monterey Jack, Muenster, Mysost (Primost), Neufchatel, Portsalut, Provolone, Romano, Roquefort, Stilton, Swiss, Tillamook, and Tilsiter.

Fruits and Vegetables

★ *Servings per day: At least*
Three (3) portions of fruits; plus
Three (3) portions of vegetables.

Estimates of portions in this Cluster include for 1 portion: 1/2 cup of cooked, canned, or dried fruits *or* 1 cup of raw fruit *or* 1 piece fresh fruit; *or*
1/2 cup of canned or cooked vegetables *or* 1 cup raw vegetables.

Fruits and vegetables contribute fiber, Vitamin A, Vitamin C, thiamine, some iron, riboflavin, and folacin. Mustard greens, collard greens, cantaloupe, carrots, kale, Swiss chard, spinach, apricots, acorn squash, and sweet potatoes are excellent sources of Vitamin A. Mustard greens, strawberries, collard greens, papaya, broccoli, cabbage, cantaloupe, cauliflower, kale, kiwi, grapefruit, Brussels sprouts, oranges, potatoes, bell peppers, and prunes are fruits and vegetables high in Vitamin C.

It is important to include "cruciferous" vegetables in your plan. They provide fiber, Vitamins A or C, and are thought to help prevent some kinds of cancers. Cruciferous vegetables are broccoli, Brussels sprouts, cabbage, cauliflower, kale, kohlrabi, mustard greens, and Swiss chard.

This double, dynamic, dynamite Cluster includes fresh, frozen, canned, cooked, raw, or dried fruits or fruit juices (fruits and juices preferably without added sugars); and raw, canned, frozen, or cooked vegetables. Include tomato and vegetable juices, tomato products such as sauce and puree, hot sauce and salsa, and salad vegetables in this Cluster.

High-fat vegetables are any buttered or creamed vegetables; vegetables with cheese; fried vegetables such as mushrooms, okra, zucchini, etc. Often pizza, spaghetti, and other tomato products and sauces contain a significant amount of fat. When grocery shopping and reading labels, select vegetables lowest in fat and sodium for better health.

> *"Does not nature produce enough simple vegetable foods to satisfy? And if not content with such simplicity can you not, by the mixture of them, produce infinite variations?"*
> —*Leonardo da Vinci*

Breads, Grains, and Cereals

This Cluster includes breads, grain products (rice, pastas, crackers, rolls, bagels), and cooked or dry unsugared cereals.

★ *Servings per day: At least four to six portions.*

For additional calories, complex carbohydrates, and fiber, add more from this Cluster.

Estimates to use for portion sizes in this Cluster are:

1 slice of bread;
1/2 cup cooked cereal, rice, or pasta;
1 cup dry cereal;
1/2 dozen crackers.

Breads, grains, and cereals are significant sources of complex carbohydrates, and provide niacin, iron, thiamine,

and in whole grains, fiber and zinc. Whole grains are whole wheats, oats, unpolished rice, barley, millet, rye, and bulgur.
—*Breads/rolls*: Whole wheat, whole grain, and enriched breads and cereals. French, Italian, sourdough, oatmeal, pita, pumpernickel, raisin, and rye breads and rolls, hard rolls, bagels, bagel chips, English muffins, Melba toast, bread sticks, corn and flour tortillas, hamburger buns, and rusk.

—*Crackers*: Any fat-free including matzoth, saltines, soda, oyster, rye wafers, graham and teddy graham crackers, Kavli, WasaBröt, Lahvosh, zwieback, rice cakes, and corn cakes.

—*Cereals and Grains*: Brown, white, or wild rice; Bulgur or Kasha (groats); dry or cooked without coconut, oils, fats, or nuts; bran cereals, oat bran; cornmeal, cornstarch; air-popped popcorn (without fat); pasta (linguini, macaroni, noodles, shells, spaghetti, etc.).

Breads, grains, and cereals which are *higher* in fat and that you may want to eliminate at your meals and snacks to reduce the fat and possible cholesterol content of your foods include:

—*High-fat breads/rolls*: Egg or cheese breads, butter or pan rolls, biscuits, croissants, cornbread, muffins, pancakes, and potato pancakes, waffles, French toast; bread stuffing, bread mixes; egg and cheese bagels; sweet rolls, doughnuts, Danish pastries, cinnamon rolls, banana, and other nut breads.

—*High-fat crackers:* corn chips, cheese crackers, other flavored crackers; Ritz®, Waverly Wafers®, seasoned rye crackers; WasaBröt with seeds; and matzoh brei.

—*High-fat cereals*: Any natural grain cereal containing coconut or nuts, trail mixes, granolas, pre-packaged pasta products (e.g., macaroni or noodles) prepared with regular cheeses or sauces, microwave popcorn, pre-popped popcorn with oil, fat, or cheese, commercial mixes for baked products containing eggs, whole milk, and fats (unsaturated, saturated or hydrogenated): e.g., cake, biscuit, brownie mixes, etc.

Some of the traditionally high-fat or high-cholesterol foods can easily be made at home and adapted for lower cholesterol or fat consumption. Replace eggs with low-cholesterol egg substitutes. Use no fats or oil in preparation or in cooking. Use non-stick frying or baking pans, or use a vegetable spray to lightly coat pans before cooking.

High Protein Foods

This Cluster includes predominantly low-fat and lean cuts of meats, fish, and poultry, some cheeses, cottage cheese, eggs, and low-fat luncheon meats.

★ *Servings per day: Maximum of five ounces; or 1-1/2 cups per day; or substitute 1/2 cup dried beans/dried peas/lentils (Cluster #1) for one (1) ounce meat* (prepared the way you will be eating the food; for instance, weigh or measure meats after preparation and cooking).

Animal proteins contribute iron, riboflavin, niacin, zinc, vitamin B_{12}, and thiamine to your diet. Animal protein sources contain saturated fats and cholesterol. The fat and cholesterol content varies with each source of protein and the area or section of the animal.

★ *Leaner meats and substitutes*

Poultry: Chicken and stewing hens, turkey, Cornish hens, game birds such as wild duck, goose, or squab without skin or fat. Ground turkey, turkey hot dogs, and luncheon meats (ham, salami, etc.) with 5% or less fat.

Fish: Fresh and frozen "fin" fish (without breading): bass, catfish, cod, flounder, gefilte, haddock, halibut, herring (uncreamed or smoked), lobster, mackerel, perch, pike, pollock, red snapper, salmon (fresh or canned in water), sardines (canned), scrod, smelt, sole, trout, tuna (fresh or packed in water), turbot, whitefish, etc.; fish canned in water or rinsed. Shellfish (fresh or canned in water): crab, lobster, and shrimp. Scallops; abalone; oysters; clams.

Veal: Lean cuts such as chops, roast or steaks.

Beef: USDA Good or Choice grades of lean beef, such as round steak, sirloin, tenderloin, filet mignon, flank steak, London broil, rump roast, chipped beef, tripe.

Pork: Lean, such as tenderloin, loin chops, roast, Boston butt, fresh, canned, cured or boiled ham, Canadian bacon.

Lamb: Loin chops, leg and arm roast.

Wild game: Venison, javelina, moose, bear, rabbit, squirrel, pheasant, quail, dove, duck (without skin), and other wild game are lower in fat and saturated fats than some cuts of beef and prime beef.

Meat substitutes: Soy protein meat substitutes. Soybean curd (tofu). 97% and 95% fat-free luncheon meat. Whole eggs (high in cholesterol) or egg whites (3 whites), and egg substitutes with fewer than 55 Calories (1/4 cup). Vegetarian baked beans. Frozen, low calorie dinners with 5 grams fat or less. Soybean curd (tofu) is moderate in vegetable fat and a piece that is 2″ x 2″ x 1 3/4″ (or 4 ounces) is equal to 1 ounce meat.

Cheeses: Cheeses which substitute for lean meats and are low in fat include: Low-fat (1% or 2%) cottage cheeses, grated Parmesan cheese. Specially prepared, low-fat diet cheeses with fat content less than 10% (e.g., Lite Line®, etc.). Skim milk mozzarella or ricotta. Pot cheese. Sapsago cheese. Jarlsburg cheese. Farmer's, baker's or hoop cheese with 10% or less fat.

Most cuts of beef and pork, and all lamb, have a moderate amount of fat, saturated fat, and cholesterol. Egg yolks, liver, heart, kidney, and sweetbreads are very high in cholesterol. Egg substitutes which are about 56-80 calories per 1/4 cup serving are moderate in fat and saturated fat.

★ *Higher-fat meats and substitutes*

Higher-fat and saturated fat cuts of beef, pork, lamb, fish, and cheeses are:

Poultry: Any poultry with skin or fried. Goose and domesticated duck. Chicken livers, paté, giblets, heart.

Fish: Any fried fish product, such as fish sticks, oil-packed tuna, sardines, caviar, fish roe.

Veal: Cutlet (ground or cubed).

Beef: Organ meats including liver, kidney, heart, sweetbreads. Fatty or heavily marbled meats, prime rib, chuck roast, T-bone and New York cut steaks; canned meat products, corned beef, brisket; "regular" ground beef or hamburger; short ribs; all-beef frankfurters; USDA prime cuts of beef, and ribs.

Pork: Blade roll; bacon, ham hocks, sausage (patties or links), spareribs, ground pork. Luncheon meats (bologna, cold cuts, frankfurters, salami, etc.)

Lamb: Patties, ground lamb.

Meat substitutes: Dried beans/dried peas/lentils cooked with pork, bacon, ham, or animal fat; refried beans.

Other: Luncheon meat, such as bologna, salami, pimento loaf, pastrami, salami, pepperoni, etc.; head cheese; 86% fat free luncheon meats; sausages such as Polish, Italian, Knockwurst, smoked, Brätwurst, liverwurst, frankfurters, and hot dogs (turkey or chicken). "Convenience" foods: packaged, frozen or canned with more than 2 grams fat per serving; "TV" dinners with more than 5 grams fat. Mexican food; Italian food. BLT sandwich. Fast food sandwiches and burgers.

Cheeses: "Regular" cheeses, such as American, Bal Paese, Blue (Bleu), Boursault, Brick, Brie, Camembert, Caraway, Caciocavallo, Cheddar, Colby, Dolfino, Edam, Feta, Fontina, Formage de chevre, Gjetost, Gorgonzola, Gouda, Greyerzer, Gruyere, Liederkranz, Liptauer, Limburger, Monterey Jack, Muenster, Mysost (Primost), Neufchatel, Portsalut, Provolone, Romano, Roquefort, Stilton, Swiss, Tillamook, Tilsiter, processed cheeses and cream cheese are high in fats and saturated fats.

Some products that are often prepared with or served with high-fat cheeses are: Mexican foods, refried beans; pizza; Italian foods; cheese soups and sauces; and dips for chips or vegetables.

★ *Fats and Oils*

For balanced nutrient intake, a minimal amount of fats or oils are needed. The fats and oils are from plant sources, and contain more unsaturated fats with fewer hydrogenated fats, and therefore have a lower amount of saturated fats than lard or butter. For this minimal amount of more unsaturated fats and oils, the following list is provided.

Limit to 3 servings or less per day in cooking, or as an addition to a food:

1 teaspoon corn, safflower, peanut, olive, or rapeseed (canola) oil; polyunsaturated margarine; *or*

2 teaspoons special mayonnaise or diet corn or safflower oil margarine; *or*

2 teaspoons French, Italian, Russian, or Vinaigrette dressings; *or*

3 tablespoons avocado or guacamole made without sour cream; *or*

Unlimited: fat-free, oil-free salad dressings, and fat-free butter substitutes (e.g., Molly McButter®).

Foods with significant amounts of saturated fats or cholesterol include: bacon, lard, or other meat drippings, chicken fat, butter, solid shortenings, hydrogenated oils, fats or margarine, diet margarine, sour cream, cream cheese, and diet cream cheese, salad dressings with mayonnaise, blue cheese or Roquefort cheese, "low calorie" salad dressings, coconut, palm or palm kernel oils, commercial garlic spreads, cocoa butter, dips for vegetables, guacamole made with sour cream.

LIFESTYLE CHANGES

POINTS TO REMEMBER

★ Eat a variety of foods from each of the five Food Clusters.
  1 Dried beans, dried peas and lentils
  2 Milk
  3 Fruits and 3 vegetables
  4 Breads, cereals, and grains
  5 (ounces) Meat

★ Increase fiber by eating legumes, raw fruits, and raw vegetables.

★ Increase complex carbohydrates by having more breads, cereals, and grains.

★ Limit High Protein (meat) portions to 5 ounces total per day.

★ Decrease fat in foods and meals.

Chapter 6
BREAKFAST, LUNCH, DINNER, AND SNACKS

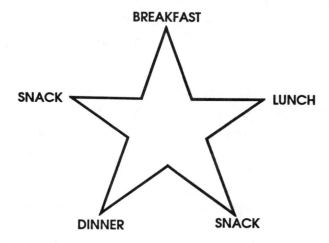

We have been undisciplined in our approach to food and meals. We may have inconvenienced others because of our self-centered desires about our "drug of choice" and eating and enjoying meals. We can evaluate our attitudes and habits about meals and change them by changing when we eat. We require food and energy throughout the day to keep us going.

Breakfast, lunch, and dinner (three "squares" a day) contain food items from at least three (3) of the five (5) different Food Clusters. **Snacks** consist of at least two (2) of the five (5) different Food Clusters.

Meals and snacks provide essential nutrients, calories, and an opportunity to heal, socialize, and work some of the Steps, especially Steps Six, Seven, Nine, Ten, and Twelve.

Some of you are probably grumbling and complaining about eating that often and *having* to have breakfast. Some of us, when abusing, were so "hung over" or feeling so bad that we couldn't eat or didn't care, and have carried that behavior and attitude into recovery. Some of us grew up in dysfunctional families, or are adult children of alcoholic or drug-abusing parents, and never learned appropriate eating behaviors. Some of us believe that "we" are different and therefore exempt from change.

In recovery, it is our choice to continue to grow and benefit from new information, attitudes, and behaviors. This is a great opportunity to let go of beliefs, attitudes, values, behaviors, and habits that are not conducive to our general good health, well-being, and sanity in recovery.

When our ideas about eating and meals come from television, there are flaws in our information and it is not adequate for day-to-day meals. Television rarely shows people truly eating. When eating is shown, it is usually the men who eat and the women who serve. Rarely do women literally "eat" in movies or television, even though they are at the meal or are providing food.

Also, television meals often depict times of emotional abuse, ridicule, derision, and contempt. In situation comedies, meals are a time to be disrespectful, insolent, or to browbeat and abuse in the name of "fun."

Television and film depictions of meals do not usually show people eating and enjoying their meals. They are more apt to show people practicing one or more addictions than to show healthy eating situations.

For improved health, meals and snacks are distributed throughout the day and at times when our bodies need additional sustenance, nutrients, calories, and care. Breakfast should be within one hour after rising; lunch is 3 to 5 hours later; dinner (supper) is 5 to 7 hours after lunch and several hours after a between-meal snack. An evening or pre-bedtime snack is within 30 minutes to 2 hours before retiring. This thought may help us to change our attitudes about our meals and when we eat:

> *Just For Today: I am an action person. I make responsible decisions about my eating habits and my actions reflect these decisions.*

Breakfast

Have breakfast within one hour after waking. For some of us this will be easy since we already get out of bed and head almost immediately for the kitchen and food. Others swear they "can't" eat breakfast, they never have, and with stubborn self-will state, "I won't start now." Eating breakfast gives us energy to start our day, improves our ability and desire to concentrate, improves our attention span, improves our attitude, and provides part of the essential nutrients our body will need for the day. People who have breakfast have a better nutrient intake than those who do not.

Examples of breakfast are:
★ Fruit or juice, and cereal with reduced-fat milk; *or*
★ Cheese crisp (flour tortilla/low fat cheese), juice; *or*
★ Juice, toast, and reduced-fat milk.

Lunch

Lunch (or our next meal about 3 to 5 hours after breakfast) includes foods from at least three of the five Food Clusters. Lunches generally are eaten between 11:30 a.m. and 1:30 p.m. If we work evening or night shifts, our "lunch-time" may be closer to midnight than noon. Whether we eat at home, "brown-bag" it, or eat out, our meal might be:
★ Sandwich with whole grain bread, low-fat lunch meat, mustard, lettuce, tomatoes, and fruit (apple); *or*
★ Chili with beans, crackers, and reduced-fat milk.

Our facilities at work or school influence what we "brown-bag" for lunch. When we have access to a refrigerator, microwave, oven, or toaster oven, we may take perishable, frozen, or reheatable foods. If our lunch stays with us at room temperature or out-of-doors, choices of foods are more restricted.

Dinner

Dinner (supper) includes at least three (3) of the five Food Clusters. Examples are:

★ Grilled or broiled fish, tossed salad, corn on the cob, garlic toast; *or*

★ Broiled or grilled chicken breast on a whole wheat bun with tomato, lettuce, onion, mustard, baked or "cowboy" beans.

Snacks

Snacks in the afternoon and later evening incorporate at least 2 of the five Food Clusters. Afternoon snacks are important; they help us keep our attitude "up" and avoid having a late afternoon slump in thinking, concentration, and activity. Some evening snacks will be after a meeting, when we go for "coffee" with our friends. Enjoy decaffeinated coffee and a light snack; avoid real or "leaded" coffee, and sugar-laden, fat-laden pies, cakes, cookies, and other pastries. Some soups, sandwiches, and appetizers are great choices for healthy, readily available evening snacks. Some examples of healthy snacks when eating out are:

★ Sandwich on rye bread (half or a whole); *or*

★ Bagel (yes, we can eat it plain) and juice; *or*

★ Cottage cheese and fruit salad; *or*

★ Vegetable soup and crackers.

Healthy snacks at home may be:

★ Popcorn, air-popped, and fresh fruit; *or*

★ Low-fat cheese and crackers (or nachos); *or*

★ Cereal and reduced fat milk; *or*

★ "Left overs" from lunch or dinner; *or*

★ Cheese crisp (quesadilla) made with low-fat cheese; *or*

★ Fresh or frozen fruit dipped in plain, fat-free yogurt: apples, oranges, berries, melons, grapefruit, bananas, peaches, pineapple, etc.

For ideas about foods to incorporate into our snacks, have one or more of the following in combination with another item from a different Food Cluster.

Fruit juices: Apple, orange, grapefruit, pineapple, grape, prune, berry, etc., or tomato juice or vegetable juice cocktail, vegetable juices with added seasonings, spices, and herbs.

Fresh fruits and vegetables: Apple wedges, bell pepper, carrot sticks, celery sticks, celery with peanut butter (old fashioned or homemade) or yogurt dip, cucumber chunks, jicama chunks, turnip slices, zucchini chunks.

Popcorn: air-popped and without fat or margarine added.

Dry cereal, unsugared, with skim milk.

Muesli: homemade with fat-free yogurt, uncooked oatmeal/ dry cereal, and fruits.

Breads and crackers: Bagel, bagel chips, bread sticks, corn or flour tortilla or baked tortilla chips, dry cereals like Cheerios®, plain bite-sized shredded wheat biscuits, graham crackers and "teddy grahams," Lavhosh, matzoh, melba toast, mini-muffins, oyster crackers, pita pocket, pretzels (preferably unsalted), rice cakes or wafers, rusks, plain rye crackers, saltine-style crackers, WasaBröt, zwieback.

Raw vegetables with hot sauce (salsa): zucchini, cucumbers, peppers, cauliflower, carrots, broccoli, celery, tomatoes, Italian squashes.

Fruit or vegetable dips made with fat-free yogurt or 1% fat cottage cheese.

"Slushies" made by blenderizing skim milk and fruit.

Carbonated beverages: diet or club soda.

Decaffeinated coffee and tea, cereal beverages (e.g., Postum).

Broth-based soups: homemade or no more than 1/2 can of commercial soups; or broth or bouillon.

Low-fat cheeses: Cottage cheese, mozzarella, pot cheese, "light" American.

Lean Meats: Turkey, ham, roast beef, 97% fat free luncheon meats.

Low-fat yogurt dip with raw vegetables or fruit.

Homemade, mashed, and seasoned *bean dip*.

Milk: 2%, 1%, skim, or buttermilk.

When we work evening shifts and sleep during the day, our meals and snacks obviously are at different times. A "dinner" may be the meal we eat when we get up; lunch may be our "dinner" meal; and "breakfast" may be the last meal we eat before retiring. We may also have two routine schedules for meals: one for the nights we work and another for the days we are off.

Other times when our meals may need to be adjusted are when we travel extensively or cross continents or oceans. These times take some very creative planning to fit into our meal and food plans in recovery. You may be adapting to different time zones, cultures, mores, activities, expectations, and feelings of acceptability.

Character "defects" can help or hinder us in recovery. Perhaps we are working to remove a character defect which occurs at or because of meals, food, or eating. The thought processes of a substance abuser are highly creative and at times downright sneaky. We have used these thought processes to abuse substances, to hide the abuse, to make excuses to others, to blame, to find fault, to avoid, and to avoid recovery. We can now use these same intricate, sometimes devilish processes to think of ways to incorporate appropriate meals and snacks into our lifestyle of recovery.

> *Just For Today: I am very satisfied with my new, balanced eating plan. My accomplishments please and delight me.*

Chapter 7
SHOPPING SMART, EATING RIGHT, EATING OUT

Make a searching and fearless food inventory of your kitchen, refrigerator, freezer, storeroom and pantry. See what you have, what you want to keep, and what you want to get rid of and not restock. Make a list of all foods that may harm you, that you want out of your life for your improved meal and eating program. Throw out foods that are detrimental to health and well-being. Continue to evaluate the foods you select and eat, and when you select inappropriate items, promptly admit it, omit, and discard them.

> *Just For Today: I am an action person. I make responsible decisions about my eating habits and my actions reflect these decisions.*

Shopping Smart

Once you know what you have in your kitchen, and before you go to the grocery store or send someone else for your shopping, *have a grocery list.* Carefully check it over to be sure all the foods you need and want are on this list. Also, check that you are not planning to purchase more of some foods than you need, and that you are not indulging someone else by buying extra "goodies." When you are shopping, do not add other foods to your grocery cart because they are on sale or tempt you. If they tempt you in the store, they will tempt you at home. When someone else is shopping for you, do not let them purchase other food items for you just because *they* think you need them.

★ **Shop after you have eaten.** If you are hungry when you go grocery shopping, you will buy more than you plan to buy, and more of the foods that are hazardous to your new eating program: sugary, salty, snack foods, and fattier foods. Most of these are not in your new eating program. Changing food habits is difficult enough without causing yourself more problems.

★ **Shop alone or with a trusted friend or relative.** There are literally hundreds of items tempting you to toss them into your grocery basket, so the fewer distractions the better. A *trusted* friend or relative is helpful since he/she may help you buy only what is on your list and avoid temptations.

★ **Purchase foods that require preparation.** Foods prepared at home are usually lower in fats, salt, sugar, and calories than foods that do not require preparation. This is an ideal way for people who enjoy cooking/baking to use their talents to enhance a new eating program. Foods that do not require preparation routinely have more fatty and sugary ingredients than a homemade version.

★ **Buy fresh fruits and vegetables in season.** Fresh fruits are more enjoyable to eat. Raw vegetables make great salads and munchies. In season, both are more economical to have and to use than frozen or canned products.

Purchase fruits and vegetables of varying degrees of ripeness. Some you can eat immediately; some will keep for later. Remember to buy enough, since others in your home will enjoy them as much as you do.

Wash, clean, and prepare raw vegetables and some fruits for munching immediately after you have put away your other groceries. Then they will be readily available for snacks and hunger attacks when you want them.

★ **Learn to read and interpret information on the labels.** Most packaged foods have ingredient and product information printed on the label of the container. This information is either required by law or offered by the food manufacturer.

Eating Right

In October 1990, Congress passed the Nutrition Labeling and Education Act. Its interpretation is in process, and changes on labels will be introduced over the next few years. The Act covers all foods regulated by the Food and Drug Administration, but does *not* cover meat and poultry products, restaurant foods, or grocery store salad and deli bars.

The Act requires food manufacturers to use readable, uniform nutrition labeling in a simple format, with standardized serving sizes and household measures. The descriptive terms "light," "low-calorie," "high-fiber," "cholesterol-free," etc., will not be allowed. Labeling of foods that make nutrient or health claims will be much more restricted. The following nutritional terms and statements can be used when the product doesn't contain other ingredient(s) which are potentially detrimental to good health:

Fiber: foods high in fiber may reduce the risk of cancer and heart disease.

Fat: A low fat diet may reduce the risk of cancer and heart disease.

Sodium: A low sodium diet may help prevent high blood pressure.

Calcium: Foods high in calcium may help prevent osteoporosis.

Labeling of 20 most commonly eaten fresh fruits, vegetables, and seafood will be voluntary. It will probably appear as signs, booklets, or "shelf talkers" near the respective sections.

In 1968, the FDA established the "U.S. RDAs" to help consumers read and interpret claims food manufacturers and processors were making. It is very likely that these will change over time as new health information is available.

Standard information on a label is:

★   common name of the product.

★   name and address of manufacturer, packer, or distributor.

★   net contents of container by weight, measure, or count.

★   a list of ingredients in descending order of quantity by weight.

Some products are not required to list ingredients since it is assumed that "everyone" knows them.   Catsup and ice cream are two of these.

Ingredients:

Ingredients are listed in descending order, from largest to smallest . Also shown are any added nutrients (vitamins and minerals).

For instance, on Nabisco Original Premium Saltine Crackers® the list of ingredients shows:

> *Enriched wheat flour (contains niacin, reduced iron, thiamine mononitrate [Vitamin B_1], riboflavin [Vitamin B_2]), animal and vegetable shortening (lard and partially hydrogenated soybean oil), salt, baking soda, malted barley flour, calcium carbonate, and yeast.*

From this list, we learn that wheat flour, enriched with vitamins and iron, is the main ingredient; yeast is the least. We also learn that lard is the animal fat and partially hardened soybean oil is the vegetable fat.   From this we can learn that the ingredients that make the flour rise (leavening agents) are baking soda and yeast.

Nutrition Information Per Serving:

Standard data and the "Nutrition Information" format contain the following:

★ Standardized serving or portion size in household measurements.

★ Servings or portions per container.

★ Calories per serving.

★ Calories from fat, protein, and carbohydrates.

★ Total fat, saturated fat, and cholesterol.

★ Sodium.

★ Sugar, fiber, protein, carbohydrates, and complex carbohydrates.

★ Protein, vitamins and minerals as percentages of the U.S. RDAs.

The U.S. RDAs required are: protein, Vitamin A, Vitamin C, the "B" vitamins of thiamine, riboflavin and niacin, and iron and calcium.

If we again look at the label of crackers we see the following:

Nutrition Information Per Serving	
Serving Size 1/2 ounce (5 crackers)	Fat .... 2 Grams
Servings Per Package 32	Polyunsaturated .... *
Calories 60	Saturated .... *
Protein .... 1 Gram	Cholesterol ... Less than 2 Milligrams
Carbohydrate .... 10 Grams	Sodium .... 180 Milligrams
*Contains Less Than 1 Gram	

Percentage of U.S. Recommended Daily Allowances (U.S. RDA)			
Protein 2	Vitamin C .... **	Riboflavin 4	Calcium 2
Vitamin A .. **	Thiamine 6	Niacin 4	Iron 4
**Contains Less Than 2% of the U.S. RDA of These Nutrients.			

The double asterisk shows nutrients of a quantity less than 2% of the U.S. RDA. This can mean 1.8% or 0%.

Serving sizes are often shown in ounces. Unless we have a food (or postage) scale to weigh out this amount, we can either guess, or follow the manufacturer statement regarding allotment that equals that weight.

Manufacturer's Address:
The name, city, and state of the manufacturer or packer is shown. You may also find additional address information such as the mailing or street address. The label may also givelocal, long distance, or "800" consumer services phone numbers. When you have additional questions or comments about the product or ingredients, you may contact the manufacturer.

Occasionally, you may want more information about ingredients because you have food allergies or sensitivities, diabetes, or other disorders that require you to be more careful about what you eat. These other health issues may be independent of your addiction but are essential for your continued recovery and prevention of relapse.

Other Product Information:
Many foods you eat don't come from grocery stores. Meals and snacks may be eaten at fast-food or chain restaurants. You may contact the "Corporate" offices of these chains and often obtain similar information about their products.

For example, McDonald's Corporation Nutrition Information Center has food and nutrition information about their products available. One booklet includes "ingredient lists" with the supplier(s), and "nutrition information per serving." Also available separately are *"Food Exchange Lists For McDonald's Restaurants* (diabetic exchanges)" and *"Calorie, Sodium, and Cholesterol Content of Foods Served at McDonald's Restaurants."* Single copies of these are available free upon request.

Other fast-food restaurants, pizza places, etc. give out similar information upon request from either local restaurants or their corporate offices. If interested, ask your local restaurant manager how you obtain this information about their eating establishment.

Just For Today: I readily make wise choices about my foods and easily support those choices.

Eating Out

One of the great American pastimes is eating out. Often after a meeting, a group will go out for "coffee," which may include a meal or a snack at a fast-food restaurant, a cafe, or a coffee shop. Other places may include a friend's or relative's, fine restaurants, potlucks, cafeterias, or picnics. You may have a choice of where you are eating and what you will eat, or it may be that "what you see is what you (may) get."

When eating out, do some advance planning. Wherever you may eat, you want it to be a healthy, enjoyable experience. There is no need to have a "stuffed stomach" and feel guilty later. Handy hints to use when you eat where you have a choice or some degree of control of what you may be eating are:

★ Make an eating plan and pre-plan, and stick to them.

★ Pre-plan your selection of your meal.

★ Eat only the amount you want.

★ Eat slowly.

★ Keep a healthy attitude.

Make your plan and pre-plan and stick to them. These will include:

★ Where, what time, with whom, what kinds of foods will be served, and are they healthy for you?

★ Know which foods fit into your plan.

★ Plan what foods to order or divide with someone else.

Order sandwiches without mayonnaise, oil, or special dressings. Order sauces, gravies, mayonnaise, etc. on the side so you can put on the amount that you want. Order lemon wedges or vinegar for your salad, or order other salad dressings on the side.

To pre-plan your selection of your meal, find out where you will be going and what will be your probable assortment from which to select. When you have an idea about what will be served, make two possible choices which will fit into your new eating style and your personal nutrition program. If you plan to divide foods with someone else, be sure that they are agreeable to what you select and to the portion they will be receiving. Remember to include a salad and a beverage.

Have an idea about the time you will eat. Your arrival time could be 15 minutes to an hour or two before you actually start eating.

Pre-planning your selection of foods is easy, regardless of the type of restaurant/facility in which you eat. Let's look at some of the different ethnic foods that are available:

Chinese/Oriental: Avoid sweet and sour foods (e.g., pork), deep fat fried foods (e.g., fried shrimp), fried rice, chow mein noodles, and other fried foods. Stir-fried foods will have extra fat, so anticipate having a higher fat meal. Order plain white rice with a vegetable/meat (fish, pork, chicken, beef) combination, clear broth soups for an appetizer, and enjoy your fortune cookie.

Mexican: Order ala carte. Choose one or two of the following regular sized items: taco, tamale, enchilada, fajita, tostado, or refried beans. Add a side order of a lettuce/tomato (vegetable) salad. Use the salsa sauce for your salad dressing and enjoy your meal. To avoid extra fat and calories, omit "chips," guacamole, sour cream, burros, burritos, chimichangas, taco salads, and extra tortillas, beans, or rice.

Other types of "ethnic" food restaurants may offer the same types of food that you are accustomed to eating at home. Always we can plan the healthiest food choices from whatever we have available. You may consider "ethnic" foods to be American, soul, Italian, Mediterranean, Greek, Polish, German, Jewish, etc. Your idea of "ethnic" foods is probably "what the other person" eats.

Salad bars and cafeterias are excellent choices since you can see all the food, how it is prepared, and how large the portion sizes are. These may be at your work place, commercial establishments, or schools. No matter where you eat, you want to be prepared for a higher risk situation.

> *Just For Today: I easily order foods in a restaurant that reflect my new, healthy eating program.*

Eat only the amount you want. Decide what and how much you will be eating and eat only those foods in the predetermined amounts. Save the rest for a "doggy bag," to share with a friend, or to have thrown out. Say "no." Be firm and be consistent when offered additional foods. "Others" who may offer you additional foods might be the server or family/friends. Someone in your group may even try to make you feel guilty for not eating everything on your plate. You can still be firm and consistent and say "no."

When you are eating, **be the most leisurely one eating**. Finish last. This will give you plenty of time to enjoy each bite, the aroma of the food, the surroundings, and, most important, the company. When you are the slowest one eating, another way to say "no" is to stop eating when everyone else is through. That way, you have "saved" a number of calories.

Throughout your meal, **maintain an attitude of gratitude**. Be grateful that you have the food to eat, money to purchase it, and friends with whom to share your meals. Remember why you are eating out and with whom. Usually people eat out to enjoy friends/family, no dishes to wash, no mess to clean up, no rush to prepare a meal, different selections, and so forth. We eat out with others to enjoy their company, share warmth, love, care, and good feelings. The purpose of the outing is to enjoy those with you, not because the food is so marvelous. It may be good and well worth eating, but the company is far more significant.

Some restaurants you might want to avoid are places like an "all-you-can-eat," or a brunch/buffet where you will be tempted to the "limit."

Good food selections are our action steps to achieve our goals of good health and vigor. Whether we eat at home or out, we can make excellent, healthy selections of the right foods for ourselves.

POINTS TO REMEMBER

★ Make decisions *before* you act.
★ Be *grateful* that you have choices to make and money with which to purchase the foods you require or desire.
★ Shop with a list, after you have eaten.
★ Buy fresh fruits and vegetables in season.
★ Learn to read and interpret labels.
★ Make responsible, healthy decisions about food, and enjoy these decisions when eating with others.

Chapter 8
SIMPLE, TASTY, APPETIZING, RESPONSIBLE, EASY

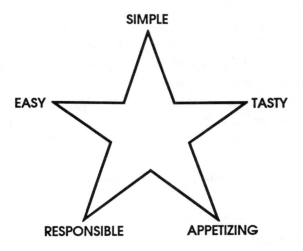

For this food guide to work better for us, it ought to be Simple, Tasty, Appealing, give us Responsibility for its start and success, and Easy to use.

Simple

Five Food Clusters (Dried Beans/Dried Peas/Lentils—Milk—Fruits and Vegetables—Breads, Grains and Cereals—High Protein clusters) to get a variety of foods, textures, and nutrients. Eat 5 times a day. Exercise no more than 5 times per week.

Keep your exercise program simple and interesting. Monitor your heart rate and wear appropriate clothes for the activity and the weather.

Tasty

How food tastes depends not only on taste acuity (intensity) but the sense of smell. The senses of taste and smell are affected by liver disease (cirrhosis), some hormonal abnormalities, high blood pressure, and nutrient deficiencies of niacin, zinc, and B_{12}. The senses of taste and/or smell may be reduced or distorted.

Foods can be as well seasoned or as mild as you choose. Sometimes, in recovery from alcoholism, excessive alcohol consumption, gastritis, or ulcers, peppers and caffeine ought to be avoided entirely to promote healing of the intestinal tract. (Also abstain from smoking and "chewing" tobaccos.)

Foods can be seasoned differently and very tastily with a variety of herbs and spices. Herbs and spices deteriorate with time, so they should be purchased in small quantities and replaced every six months or so for the fullest and best flavor. A creative way to have fresh herbs and spices is to grow your own either indoors or out.

Appealing

Appetizing food is pleasant to look at and smells inviting. Color and texture add to eye appeal. Add garnishes to plates or serving dishes. Arrange foods in a pleasing, artistic way. If you don't know how, look in women's magazines for food displays or go to buffets or cafeterias to see how it is done on a large scale. Have different colors of food at each meal. Use different colored vegetables, starches, and meats. Hot, cooked foods have more aromas than do cold foods.

Meals and food are more appealing when in a pleasant atmosphere. Allow 45 minutes to an hour for the evening meal and plan to eat with the family, if there is one. At home, turn off the television and play soft, slow music. Use place mats or table cloths. "Dine" by candlelight.

Have a *fun* exercise plan and program. Do the activities you enjoy with people you enjoy.

Responsible

Accept and take full responsibility for the foods and beverages you put into your mouth, and your interactions with others in a meal setting or eating circumstance. Making "living" amends is part of our responsibilities in recovery.

Meals are an ideal time and place to make necessary "living" amends (Step Ten) to those close to us whom we harmed. Perhaps we skipped meals, ridiculed or were abusive to the cook or cooking, tyrannized, bullied, or yelled at (or worse) our spouse, children, meal companions, or servers. Maybe we didn't prepare adequate, appropriate meals for our family. We can, over time, make amends for our selfish and hurtful behavior surrounding meals and food choices.

When exercising, be safe and responsible. Keep your pulse rate within your target heart rate zone. (See page 85 for information.)

Easy

Emphasize and select foods that are obvious for good and improved health and simple to prepare, select, and obtain. Remember the simple guidelines presented here. Do it *one day at a time.*

> *Just for Today: I will make responsible choices about food. I will keep my meals and snacks simple, pleasant, and easy for myself and others.*

Chapter 9
MAINTAIN A HEALTHY WEIGHT

"Flab is Drab!" and we want to be a healthy, vibrant person. Achieving and maintaining our best weight is one goal in changing our eating habits for better health. You may be at your best weight. Deciding your "best" body weight depends on your sex and your height compared with your weight. To calculate your best weight:

For women:

Add 5 pounds to your base weight for each inch over 5 feet tall.

  Base: __100__
  Add: 5 pounds: _____ for each inch over 5 feet
  Best weight: _____

If you are shorter than 5 feet, deduct 5 pounds for each inch less than 5 feet. If you have a large frame, add 5 pounds. Deduct 5 pounds for a small frame.

For men:

Add 6 pounds to your base weight for each inch over 5 feet tall.

  Base: __106__
  Add: 6 pounds _____ for each inch over 5 feet
  Best weight: _____

Add 10 pounds for a large frame. Deduct 10 pounds for a small frame.

This is a general idea of your best weight. Now look in the mirror. Do you sag or "flab" in the wrong places? When you jump up and down, do you jiggle and bounce in places where you are not supposed to jiggle or bounce? Can you "pinch more than an inch" at your waist line? Do you weigh what you weighed when you were 22 years old?

> ***Just For Today:*** *I have stopped looking for ways to lose or gain weight. I have simply started to do it.*

Perhaps you are significantly underweight. Do your bones "stick out?" Are you more than 10% *under* the weight calculated above? Do your clothes hang on you? Have people told you you're too thin? Do you avoid eating in the presence of other people? Do you constantly feel full?

People who are too thin often do not recognize this. Underweight persons may benefit from the advice of a professional counselor who works in the areas of eating disorders, anorexia, bulimia, and child abuse.

Our weight affects our self-image, our self-esteem, our appearance, how old we look, how we fit into our clothes, our health, medical problems, or potential medical problems. We may have gained weight in early recovery as a reaction to the absence of our drug(s)-of-choice, to improved eating habits, and to enriched taste and enjoyment of foods. Or we may have lost weight as a reaction to our recovery and grieving our losses, and needed to find an alternative substance to abuse so we could continue to "hide" from the reality of our world and intimate relationships.

We may now want to lose or gain weight because of our desire to be healthier, to look better and feel better, for another person in our life, or because our doctor, spouse, or significant other may desire it. As with any other lifestyle change, we will always be more successful when we lose or gain weight for ourselves and our own reasons.

When we start a program to change our eating habits, we evaluate (inventory) where we are now and decide where we will be when we have accomplished our goal(s).

★ My weight goal is: _____.
★ My current weight?_____(on the scale today)
★ How much will I lose/gain? _____
★ How long will it take for me to (average pounds per week):
    lose this weight? _____ (goal is 1/2 to 2 pounds)
    gain this weight? _____ (goal is 1/4 to 3/4 pounds)
★ What size clothes do I plan to wear when I achieve this weight goal? _____
★ What size clothes do I wear now?_____
★ What health advantages are there at a lower/higher weight?_____
★ What are the family/social benefits of weighing less/more?_____

Once we have a very clear view of our goals in weight loss/gain, it is much easier and is more lasting once achieved.

You have established some of the goals that you wish to attain as you lose or gain weight. People usually have several levels of goals and interests. Let's look at some of our other interests that may interfere with weight change and changed eating habits.

Complete a searching and fearless inventory about your food and eating habits. This may best be done by keeping a Food Diary for 5 to 10 consecutive days (including a weekend and your "normal" routine). Evaluate the following:

★ Who will help you?
★ Who may interfere with or tempt you?
★ Where will it be easier for you to follow a different eating program?
★ What activities may hinder a new eating program?
★ What activities will help you in a new eating program?
★ What disadvantages are there for you to eat better?
★ What disadvantages are there for you to change weight?
★ What are your fears and apprehensions about eating healthier?

★ What are your fears and apprehensions about weight change?

You have reviewed some of the helps and hindrances you will have to successful and continued weight change. The more honest you are in answering these questions, the more successful will be your program to change your eating habits and your weight.

People, places, and things influence, help, or hinder our weight loss and different, improved nutrition habits. *People* may be our family (either family of origin or of choice), peers, friends, sponsor, counselor, relatives, business associates, and so forth. *We* may be a great source of help or hindrance in our own weight loss and change of eating habits.

Places that affect eating and nutrition include our favorite restaurants, our car, office, home, kitchen, bathroom, attendance at meetings, and our favorite time to eat.

Things that affect eating and nutrition include meetings, "belly button" and program birthdays (ours and others), holidays, weddings, funerals, christenings, bar and bat mitzvahs, graduations, travel, office parties, school parties, vacations, "feast" days like Thanksgiving, Christmas, Easter, Rosh Hoshanah, Yom Kippur, Hanukkah, or Passover.

Other *things* that will affect our weight are our emotional attachments to food, and our ideas regarding the taste, flavor, and "power" of some foods. These ideas may have to do with the healing nature, sexual enhancment, or soothing qualities of foods.

We may be an excellent cook, or have a "sweet tooth." We may need to feed others and cook for them. We may love to bake, eat out most of the time, or eat when bored, upset, or depressed. Which of these may help you and which of these may hinder you depends on them and you.

> *Just For Today: I easily discard my unrealistic beliefs about weight change.*

POINTS TO REMEMBER

★ Wherever you want to lose (gain) the most is where you will lose (gain) last. If you want to lose (gain) weight in your hips, thighs, front, back, ankles, etc. those are the areas that you will lose (gain) the last.

★ You rarely lose (gain) weight in proportion to the amount of, or lack of, hunger.

★ Men always lose or gain weight faster than women. When food and nutrition parameters are equal, men will lose or gain at least twice as rapidly as women.

★ You will reach a major weight plateau after 3 months of rigorous changes in eating habits and weight. This time period will be the "make" or "break" point of your changes and success.

★ It will take *one year* to see what kind of changes need to be more rigorous and which activities might be eliminated. We experience the events and holidays that occur with food.

★ It takes *four years* to successfully achieve and maintain a new eating habit and style, even though we may have lost or gained weight in less than a quarter of that time. *Our image of ourselves* changes slower than our weight.

★ Your rate of weight change will depend on your age, sex, height, weight, level of activity and exercise, your metabolism, how often you have lost or gained weight in the past, how much you lost the last time, how much of it you regained, how long it took to regain the weight, and how much more you added. You cannot compare yourself and your weight change with anyone else's, or even with your own previous experiences.

> ***Just For Today:*** *My new eating program includes a variety of foods, several meals and snacks a day, and a variety of textures, flavors, and preparation times.*

Chapter 10
HINTS FOR SUCCESSFUL WEIGHT CHANGE

For awhile we need to weigh and measure our foods until we realize the size of portions. This takes about 7 to 10 days. Keep a small food scale, measuring cups, and measuring spoons in the kitchen. Measurements are given in level amounts or even quantities (ounces). Use the minimum or maximum quantities in the five Food Clusters for Dried Beans/Dried Peas/Lentils, Milk, Fruits and Vegetables, Breads, Grains and Cereals, and High Protein foods to give you an idea of appropriate portion sizes for weight loss. Use portion sizes presented and measure (or weigh) very accurately. A "bit" over or a "tad" under makes a difference to your body since your body is measuring and using the calories in these "bits" and "tads."

You rarely lose weight as fast as you wish or you may not lose the inches where you want to initially. With weight loss, your fat tissue becomes smaller in some areas faster than others. As you continue to lose weight and maintain it, fat from other parts of your body becomes smaller and fat distribution changes.

Factors which affect permanent weight change are:
* ★ Quality of weight change.
* ★ Speed of weight change.
* ★ Length of time to change weight.
* ★ What affects your weight, your eating habits, and your activities.

★ Who affects what you eat and when.
★ Why you eat the way you do.
★ When you eat.
★ Where you eat.
★ How much you eat and how the foods are prepared.
★ Your food plan and program.
★ Buying and storing foods.
★ Eating away from home.
★ Foods, nutrients, and your needs.
★ What you say to yourself that will help you lose weight.
★ Cooking hints and ideas.
★ Plateaus.
★ Holidays, special occasions, and parties.

You have heard various theories of weight loss and why YOU cannot lose weight as readily or easily as the next person. Our metabolism affects our potential weight and weight loss. Exercise and activity will have an effect on weight. Obviously what we eat (time, quality, and quantity) affects our weight and weight goals. Our attitude has an effect on these three components. Weight loss, gain, and control is very much like a pyramid: the top is your *attitude*, with the three base corners being 1) *food and beverage* consumption (calories, protein, fat, carbohydrate, vitamins, minerals, fiber, and water); 2) *activity and exercise* levels; and 3) your *metabolism* now and as you change your nutritional intake and exercise habits.

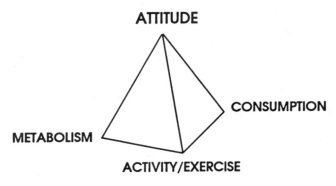

Calories are the cunning, baffling, and powerful enemy of weight loss. However, everybody needs calories to maintain body temperature and many bodily functions. Calories provide fuel for cells and the "work" of the body. Excess calories are stored as fat tissue. This is exactly what we want to get rid of. In order to do this and force your body to lose fat tissue mass, you need to reduce the calories that you put into your mouth to a level below what your body uses for energy, maintenance of body functions, and body temperature. This forces your body to dip into its reserve supply of fuel, stored fat tissue.

In addition to calories, we need *protein* in an amount that will replace body tissues as needed. We also need *carbohydrates, complex carbohydrates, some fat, fiber, vitamins, minerals, and water*. The strategies that have been devised to help with weight loss include amounts of carbohydrates, complex carbohydrates, protein, fat, and fiber for the average person. You may need slightly greater or lesser amounts of protein or fiber than is recommended.

Each time you eat, mark down the reasons that you are eating. (Refer to the Emotions Chart, p. 111.) You may have several different reasons each time you eat. You may be tired, hungry, bored, upset, or mad about something that happened. You would then mark the row for each of these feelings and reasons to eat under that day's column heading. Do this for each time you eat for the next week. Over that period, you will be finding out what triggers you to eat the most frequently. When we know what triggers us to eat, we will become more in control of our eating habits, and deal with the emotions in an appropriate way.

POINTS TO REMEMBER

★ Attitude is the key to success of our weight loss program.

★ Calories are necessary for our survival, but an overabundance of calories is stored as fat tissue.

★ Finding out why we eat and dealing with those emotions in ways other than eating is important for our well-being and health.

★ Making positive statements out loud to ourselves improves our outlook on our power and our abilities.

Your Body, Your Fat

How did you become overweight? How long have you been overweight? How many times have you tried to lose weight before? What were the obstacles to this weight loss before? Does it make a difference to your weight loss program this time?

There are many reasons people are overweight. These reasons are either physiological (glandular, metabolic, genetic, number of fat cells) or psychosocial (family function or dysfunction, self-esteem).

Family function or dysfunction may have caused some of your overweight. Our role within the family may have been a big part of this excessive weight. Food may have been used as a reward system, a pacifier, or as a mechanism to nurture and show love. Other psychological problems (depression, anxiety, etc.) may have caused the initial weight gain.

Whatever the cause of excess weight, the remedies are very similar: reduce calories eaten and/or increase calories burned (exercise). Sounds simple, right? It isn't quite that easy to accomplish. As discussed earlier, our attitude will have a definite effect on the outcome of any changes in exercise or eating habits we make.

The influence that physical problems may have on weight loss will be to slow it down as compared to a more "normal" person. This slower rate of weight loss may occur with those persons who became overweight because of a secondary cause (e.g., illness).

Some people were reared in families that used food as a reward system, for loving and as a means of pacifying others or themselves. This may cause other difficulties in losing weight. Adults who were sexually abused as children frequently develop eating disorders as a coping mechanism for survival. Coming to terms with this abuse and working through the pain and grief is necessary for long-term weight change and improved eating habits.

Each person will lose weight differently and will overcome different obstacles on their way toward lower weight. Our *attitude* is the one overriding factor that will determine our success and our loss in pounds.

Plateaus

Eventually every person who is losing weight reaches a plateau or stays at the same weight for a time. Even if we have been diligent and faithful to our new eating program, we reach a point where our weight is stable and has not gone down as we had hoped. We may also have gained a pound or two and be very discouraged, since we have been doing exactly all the right things.

Plateaus or stabilization are a normal part of losing weight. They are caused by a metabolic adjustment in your body to fat tissue loss. Keep on your weight loss plan with your new eating program and eventually your weight will start to drop again. Some plateaus are longer than others. Your plateau ought not last more that 5 days IF you have been very careful about your eating program and your other efforts to lose weight.

What you say to yourself during a plateau is important to keep your spirits up, your attitude good, and your ability to see your achievements realistically.

POINTS TO REMEMBER

★ Keep your attitude in the right place.
★ Exercise.
★ Plateaus happen; they go as readily as they come.

We are becoming more aware of why we eat, the emotions that trigger eating attacks, and we can overcome urges to overeat and overindulge. We may have rearranged the kitchen, have congenial, comfortable places in which to eat, have a pleasant atmosphere when we eat, are keeping our food records when necessary, and are eating differently than before.

One aspect of a good eating program is to enjoy the foods we eat. How we cook, season, and offer food has much to do with the satisfaction of eating. Cooking is a big part of eating and a part of the reason why many people are overweight. Being around food constantly (shopping, cooking, cleaning-up, etc.) is very tempting to even the hardiest person. We may want to change some of the times we are "interacting" with foods and food preparation.

You can be as creative as you want in who does what and how often. If you live alone, you may wish to share some of your groceries with a friend, sponsor, or neighbor who also lives alone. Perishable foods (e.g., lettuce, cabbage, celery, etc.) which may spoil before you eat them divide easily. You could share duties with a friend or neighbor; you do the shopping and he/she does the cooking. There are as many ways to share duties as there are duties to be shared.

You have changed your cooking techniques somewhat. You have learned to cook without oils, fats, lard, and butter. You have had salads without a lot of salad dressing. You are inventive and creative about mixing dishes and combining foods into tasty dishes and meals. Perhaps you have some really great recipe ideas you have shared with your friends or neighbors and will pass on to others.

Some interesting ideas may be making salsa for a zesty low calorie salad dressing, or using a red, flavored, sugar-free gelatin dessert in a chilled cranberry relish gelatin salad for holiday fare.

What we eat is what nourishes our body and our cells. What we eat and drink are part of our body's "life support" system. Food and fluids keep us alive and going in this world. Food was designed to be attractive, smell good, and taste pleasant to guarantee that people would not starve to death.

Calories are the form of energy that our body uses to keep warm (maintain body temperature), keep our cells functioning, and thereby keep us functioning and active. Excessive calorie (carbohydrate, fat, protein, alcohol) intake will result in fat storage and weight gain.

> *Just for Today: I seek to eat food on nutritional terms, just as I seek to live life on life's terms.*

Chapter 11

THE PRACTICE OF EXERCISE IN RECOVERY
Easy Does It, but Do It!

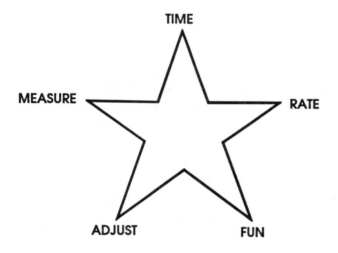

Exercise has a number of physical and psychological benefits. It maintains your muscle mass, improves your muscle tone, strengthens your heart, improves your circulation, increases your stamina, improves your appearance and shapeliness, strengthens your bones and ligaments, aids with weight loss or weight maintenance, improves your attitude toward life's ups and downs, improves self-esteem, and gives you a feeling of accomplishment. Exercise helps use calories that may normally be stored as extra fat tissue. When done correctly, exercise decreases our appetite and our desire to eat for several hours afterwards.

When we don't exercise, we tend to have flabby muscles, shortness of breath during routine physical activity, and difficulty in maintaining our best body weight. If you are not accustomed to exercise, gradually increase your exercise periods into extended workouts.

A general rule is to check with your doctor before initiating any exercise program and regarding any existing health problems which may influence the amount or type of exercise you safely can do. If you are 35 or older, have a medical examination before you **significantly** increase your exercise habits.

Select the type of cardiovascular conditioning exercise you want to do. Aerobic exercises are *rhythmic, repetitive, and filled with motion* (and sometimes emotion). Aerobic exercises include continuous, rhythmic calisthenics and dancing, walking, race walking, jogging, running, cycling, swimming (breast stroke), skipping rope, climbing stairs, rowing, and cross-country skiing. When done **continuously and rapidly** for a time, mopping or scrubbing floors, cleaning windows or vacuuming, carrying golf clubs, singles tennis, ice or roller skating, competitive handball, racquetball or squash, volleyball, badminton, or table tennis can be aerobic exercises. Muscle "bulking" exercises are not usually aerobic nor do they contribute to cardiovascular conditioning.

Some people prefer to exercise alone or in the confinement of their own homes. These kinds of exercises might be stationary cycling, using other home equipment, jogging, walking, or rowing. Others will prefer to be in a group. Group activities might include dancing, joining an exercise or aerobic class or health club, playing individual tennis, racquetball, etc. You meet interesting and fascinating people when you exercise, whether you do so in a group or while you are walking around your neighborhood.

★ **Select an aerobic exercise that will improve your cardiovascular (heart and lung) conditioning and stamina.** Exercises that are rhythmic, repetitive, and increase your heart rate to a target training rate (enough activity to increase fitness without being unsafe) for at least 20 minutes are classified as aerobic.

Determine your heart rate by counting your pulse for 15 seconds and then multiplying by four to obtain a one minute reading. Your pulse is easiest to find 1-2 inches up your inner arm from the wrist on the thumb side and just outside your tendon. Use one or two of your fingers, not your thumb, to monitor your pulse. Another place to determine your pulse rate is your carotid artery, located to the outside of your Adam's apple. Your resting pulse rate is an indicator of your general physical condition; the higher this rate, the poorer your general physical condition.

To determine your best "training" or target heart rate, use the following formula:

220 minus your current age = your maximum heart rate

220 - _____(age) = _____ maximum heart rate

maximum rate times 60-85% equals your target heart rate

_____ X .6 (or .7 or .85) = _____target heart rate

Or you can use the following as an index to a fifteen second pulse range:

AGE (years)	60-85% RATE	15 SECONDS
20	120-170	30-42
25	117-165	29-41
30	114-162	28-40
35	111-157	27-39
40	108-153	27-38
45	105-149	26-37
50	102-145	25-36
55	99-140	25-35
60	96-136	24-34
65	93-132	23-33
70	90-128	22-32
75	87-123	22-31
80	84-119	21-30

A heart rate below 60% of maximum is not adequate to improve cardiovascular conditioning; also, a rate above 85% adds little benefit to cardiovascular and muscle conditioning.

This "target heart rate" is your aim for 20 minutes of your exercise period. As your physical conditioning improves, the *intensity* of your exercise workouts increases to maintain your heart rate at that level. Also, in time, your resting heart rate will decrease. Generally, the higher your *resting* heart rate, the more physically unfit you are.

Monitoring our heart rate is important since ambient temperatures, humidity, group or individual attitudes can give us a false sense about the intensity of our specific workout. How much we sweat is not an indicator of the benefits of our exercise session.

★ **Keep it simple!** Select an exercise that you will consistently enjoy, that uses long (leg) muscles and the same muscles, and that you will do for a time. Think about your preferences. Do you want an exercise that you can do whenever you want and alone? Do you want to be in a group? Do you sometimes want to be with others and sometimes be alone when exercising? Cycling, walking, race walking, jogging, cross-country skiing are some of the exercises that can be done alone or with others. Do you want an indoor or outdoor exercise? What will you do consistently for weeks, months, and years that you can incorporate into your lifestyle now and if it changes?

Walking is a very easy, less physiologically stressful and forceful exercise, and doesn't require expensive equipment or clothes. Walking exercises the long muscles in a rhythmic, repetitive manner. It can be done in many kinds of weather, indoors or outdoors, alone or with someone. In extremely inclement conditions, walking can be done in a shopping mall, hallway, barn, covered walkway, underground tunnel, sports arena, or airport terminal. Dancing, when **continuously and rhythmically** done for 30 minutes or more, can be aerobic.

★ **Check with your doctor regarding your current health status and your choice of exercises.** A physical examination may be part of your personal "inventory." If you are 35 or older, have a medical exam before you significantly increase your exercise habits. For men over 35 years, there is a 10-fold increase in hidden heart disease. Some existing health problems may lessen the amount or type of exercise you can do safely. Abnormal heart rhythms, arthritis, asthma, gout, transient dizziness, high blood pressure, glaucoma, previous injuries, and obesity are among the health conditions which may limit or alter choices of healthy, safe exercises for you. Discuss your choices of exercise with your physician and adhere to his/her advice. Your physician may wish to administer tests including serum cholesterol and triglyceride levels, and an EKG (electrocardiogram) before he/she makes his/her decision.

★ **Get appropriate clothing or gear suitable for your particular exercise.** Once you have determined your "exercise of choice," you need to have the correct equipment or clothes to prevent any injuries. It is extremely important to have a very good pair of shoes designed for the exercise you have selected. High top shoes help to prevent sprains in some exercises. Other equipment or gear you may need include a helmet or other protective headgear, socks, and gloves. Choose under- and outer-wear which are comfortable, suitable for weather conditions, the proper size, and fit the way they should without rubbing, chafing, tightness, or looseness.

★ **Develop a schedule or plan on where and when you will be exercising.** Plan your schedule so that you have the time to exercise with time also to warm-up, cool-down, and change clothes before your next activity. Your schedule may change with changing weather patterns or the season of the year. Cross-country skiing or swimming may be such exercises.

Schedule your exercise periods so that they don't interfere with your meals, snacks, or sleep. Exercise not only suppresses your appetite temporarily but can kindle your energy level so that you are more alert and wide-awake. It may therefore interfere with your sleep if done late enough at night.

For your exercise regimen to yield the most return:

★ It lasts for 30 to 45 minutes: this includes 5 minute warm-up and 5 minute cool-down periods and at least 20 minutes of exercise at your target heart rate.

★ Is at least three (3) non-consecutive days of the week. Take at least 2 days off per week to rest and rejuvenate your muscles. Becoming obsessive-compulsive about exercising may become a "substitute substance" in your addictive process.

★ Changes once a month. Change either the rate, intensity, or distance to keep improving your physical condition. This helps to keep your target heart rate between 60% to 85% of maximum on a consistent basis.

★ **Set some reasonable, realistic goals regarding your selected exercise program.** You may have weight, size, shape or food/eating goals. You may have personal achievement goals of time, distance, event, level of proficiency, or size. You may set a goal to complete a marathon or 5K race next year, to lose 30 pounds this year, to wear that "perfect size" (again), to fit into the clothes that you already have but that don't quite "look right," to feel better and be able to move with greater agility.

Write your goals down, when you started and when you expect to accomplish these goals. Be realistic about your timetable; as you get older (or more mature) it takes longer to condition your body and you may never be able to attain your best personal record achieved when a young adult or teen. Whatever your goal, do an inventory of your physical status. Note your level of proficiency and size/shape/weight before you get really started. For measures of body size/shape, measure your biceps, neck, chest, waist, hips, thighs, calves, and ankles, and weigh yourself. For a woman, take bust as well as chest measurements.

When one of our goals is weight reduction, aerobic exercises help to maintain our muscle mass as we lose weight. The pounds we lose will reflect greater fat tissue loss instead of greater protein/muscle mass loss.

Exercise may require that we eat more calories to maintain our weight. Add extra calories by eating more complex carbohydrates (dried beans and dried peas, grains, starches and breads) and fruits. Additional amounts of high protein foods or protein supplements are not required to build additional muscle mass. Despite the "hype" regarding the need for extra protein to build muscles, this extra amount is around 10% more protein than normal physiologic needs (as you calculated earlier). With the extra complex carbohydrates of grains, dried beans, dried peas and breads eaten for calories there is sufficient additional protein.

To maintain electrolyte balance, additional potassium may be obtained by eating more vegetables, and fruits. Potatoes, bananas, mushrooms, and oranges and citrus fruits are high in potassium. Drinking adequate amounts of fluid and water is recommended. Drink at least 1 quart of water within 3 hours after an extended workout or heavy perspiration. Additional sodium or salt is unnecessary unless your physician advises that you eat "salty" foods. Several decades ago, it was a popular practice to take salt tablets for intensive exercises. This has been shown to be unnecessary and, in some cases, harmful.

Muscle mass or bulk development, and improved physical conditioning are functions of the type of exercise completed, skeletal structure, heredity (genetic and metabolic characteristics), nutritional status, sleep and rest habits, age (physiologic and chronologic), handicaps and injuries, previous level of muscle development, attitude, and length of time in recovery.

★ **The best exercise programs are those that are *fun* and *safe*.** To prevent injuries, wear appropriate clothing, and take the time to warm up and cool off for at least 5 minutes both before and after your exercise session.

"No pain, no gain!" is a myth and can result in serious bodily harm. Injuries may interfere with, stop, or prevent continuation of your selected exercise plan. If you suffer any injury, you may need to put your exercise plan on hold until you heal; you may need to see a physician; or you may need to slow down your particular exercise schedule.

Injuries that we can reasonably treat ourselves are muscle cramps, charley horses, shin splints, shortness of breath, insomnia, prolonged fatigue, and nausea or vomiting after exercise. Some of these symptoms suggest that we have exercised obsessively/compulsively (too vigorously or too intensely) without appropriate warm-up and cool down periods. For sprains that you treat at home, remember to use the RICE acronym.

Rest: rest your body and the sprain;

Ice: immediately put ice on it;

Compression: "compress" or wrap the sprained area with an expandable bandage wrap. To prevent additional damage, do not wrap too tightly; and,

Elevate: raise the injured limb. When you sprain your ankle, keep your foot elevated slightly above or at hip level when seated.

Injuries that *immediately require you to stop* your exercise program and possibly see your physician include chest pain; abnormal, irregular heart rhythms; fainting; confusion or disorientation; cold sweats; and, dizziness. Chest pains, radiating pains in your shoulder, upper arm, or throat are symptoms that require immediate attention from your physician.

After all these "cautions," go forth and enjoy yourself, exercise in health, and watch yourself develop a well-toned body and a more positive outlook on life.

POINTS TO REMEMBER

★ **Fun:** Pick an exercise you enjoy and in which your long muscles are used!

★ **Time:** Do it 3 to 5 times per week 30 to 45 minutes each session!

★ **Rate:** Maintain your target heart rate for at least 20 minutes!

★ **Adjust:** Change your exercise intensity each month!

★ **Measure:** Monitor your heart rate, weight, and health improvement gains as recommended.

Chapter 12
EMOTIONS AND FOOD
Hungry, Angry, Lonely, Tired, and Thirsty

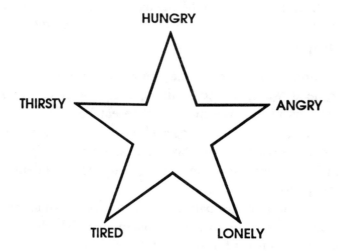

Food provides nutrients for our physical life and growth. The rhythmic activity of chewing is comforting and soothing. This nurturing sensation occurs regardless of the calories in the food. Celery or raw carrots are equally as beneficial in achieving feelings of comfort as potato chips, without the extra calories and fat. Food is not a magic potion that makes life happy, joyous, or free. Food is food; it is the form of our nutrients.

When food is used to provide comfort, escape from pain, for hiding behind, or as a display of power or wealth, it is being used improperly. When emotions, desires, and imagination enter into eating and food, sanity leaves. Flavors are glorified; sensations are justified; and mood swings can occur. Misplaced emotions and imagination about food will always win over self-will and wisdom. (See Emotions Chart, p. 111.)

A reason for this Cluster or division is to avoid the "whammies" and pain that goes with being too hungry, angry, lonely, tired, and thirsty.

Spacing meals and snacks will help avoid the feelings of cravings, hunger, and deprivation throughout the day. This also helps keep your energy level higher, your ability to concentrate and focus on the present easier, avoid tiredness, and manage and direct your "Anger" level for positive actions.

Hungry

Feeling the need to eat may be a response to loneliness, anger, need, want, stuffed feelings, using food as a tranquilizer, and comfort. We may want to eat because someone suggested it, we were watching a television commercial, or we went to the movies and we *always* had snacks. Perhaps we are eating to "please" someone else (being codependent or a "people pleaser").

Hunger and hunger pangs are often feelings of an honest "gut" level response to a circumstance in which we feel apprehensive, uncomfortable, or unsafe. Your "gut" does do flip-flops, move around and respond physiologically to feelings of "fright" or "flight." This may be a warning for real or imagined hazards. It may also be a response to being thirsty or tired.

To avoid being truly hungry there are three meals and two snacks for our eating enjoyment and pleasure. They will keep us away from unhealthy mood changes, eating behaviors, and nutritionally empty foods. The snacks help maintain balanced blood sugars and nutrient intake when the body is more apt to need them.

Just For Today: I eat five times a day to keep physically healthy. My spiritual program in recovery is affected when I am too hungry.

Angry

Sometimes food helps us feel more "mellow" and resist feeling the need to return to our substance abuse practices or our codependent, manipulative behavior. We may also be using food as a substitute substance to stuff our feelings and not deal with the emotion or real anger and rage that we may have.

There are ways to release anger without harmful effects to ourselves or others. Identifying this emotion is paramount before we can release and vent it. Evaluate your desire to eat, your choices when you eat, and other health habits to ascertain if your "feeling" has a physiological basis or is strictly an emotional reaction (current or delayed).

Just For Today: I eat before I feel any physical symptoms of hunger, anger, or discouragement. I know my anger can cause resentments which are harmful to my serenity and my program.

Lonely

Food can "buy" friendship, sex, love, and care. Food in history has brought wealth and fame to people. Its lack has destroyed armies. The saying, "The way to a man's heart is through his stomach" is not an old wives' tale.

Eating and meals can be social events, associated with nurturing and caring. Many business and professional meetings, events, and life are planned around and involve food. When people celebrate promotions, anniversaries, raises, weddings, birthdays, and "rites of passage," there is usually food. Incorporate some of your eating activities to coincide with or enhance your social needs and social interactions. However, remember your needs and the needs you are fulfilling when you interact with others and food.

The 12 Steps which could involve or revolve around some socialization and food are Steps Five, Nine, Ten, and Twelve. Eating sensibly in a positive, nurturing atmosphere can help us work these steps in recovery and sanity. Additionally we can work these steps in our family to overcome some of the dysfunctional behaviors that occurred when we were in our drinking/abusing stages. When alcoholism and drug abuse is active within a family system, there are emotional and possibly physical abuses to all members of the family and social group regardless of position, age, or sex.

Meals and eating occasions with our family, peers, business associates, and friends are ideal opportunities to work Steps Nine, Ten, and Twelve each day.

> *Just For Today: I realize my loneliness is potentially harmful to my recovery and improved health. When lonely, I go to more meetings and call my sponsor.*

Tired

Learn to recognize the difference between "tired" and "hungry." Be realistic! Tune into your needs and what your body is saying to you. When tired, take a nap, change what you are doing, go to bed earlier, avoid overdosing on caffeine or other stimulants to keep you alert. Learn what your body is telling you. Admit what your body is saying. Listen to your body! Act on the positive, healthy news your body gives you!

> *Just For Today: When I am tired, I am more apt to want to abuse substances to keep me going. I take a break from what I am doing and rest when I am tired.*

Thirsty

Drink at least ten (10) eight (8) ounce glasses of *water* each day (80 ounces or 2.5 quarts). This helps maintain electrolyte balance. Fluid is lost through skin and lungs (respiration), urine and feces. As we get older, we do not recognize our need for fluids as readily as we did when younger. Fluids help to keep your body functions and organs working properly.

Fluids other than "plain" water are juices, club soda, seltzer waters, and mineral waters. If your water has a bad taste to you, you may wish to invest in bottled water. In parts of the country where there is intensive water treatment, sometimes chilling your water or letting it sit overnight improves its taste and acceptability. However, complaints about the water flavor may be an indication of a general lack of content with your life.

> *Just for Today: I need fluids throughout the day. I gladly drink large amounts of water with my meals and in between meals for my improved health.*

Chapter 13
ATTITUDES, BELIEFS, AND HABITS
POWER OF FOOD AND SELF-POWER

To be truly adept at keeping up with a new, healthier eating program, it will take a cycle of one year to live through and learn from the events that happen to you. There are birthdays (yours and others), and other celebrations which you attend and eat.

Food is a national pastime. It is a hobby and a reason to get together. It takes about a year to go through the cycle of events that happen to us and that have tempting foods available. What we do about these occasions can be beneficial to our new, healthier eating program. We only live one occasion at a time and we learn from each occasion. We apply this knowledge to the next occasion and to the similar occasion next year.

POWER OF FOOD

You are undoubtedly aware that food has power. Food "buys" good behavior from children. It "buys" love and affection from some friends or family members. Food is power to the giver and to the receiver when it is used as a substitute for love, affection, warmth, praise, rewards, and congratulations, or when it is used to bribe, punish, procure obedience, gratitude, sex, or money.

We have looked into some of the ways we used food with our family and friends. We discovered that not all is what it had appeared to be. We have had pressures to eat and to eat foods that we did not want to eat. We undoubtedly saw the emotional energy consumed in using the power of food to control and see it now to change our eating style and habits.

Resolving the pressures to eat is time-consuming and requires mental alertness to the occasions and the people who try to tempt us. People may try to pressure us to eat unwanted foods for a variety of reasons.

Some people around us may feel uncomfortable when we are not eating exactly what they are eating. They may also feel that what we are eating is not enough for us and that we may be doing harm to our body.

Sometimes people are jealous of our success at changing our eating habits and try to undermine that success. They may be envious of our efforts at changing and eating better and wish to derail our continued efforts.

Just For Today: I have the courage and wisdom to change and become healthier.

Besides being jealous of our success and effort, sometimes people are afraid of our personal success and power. They fear that successes and self-empowerment to change our eating habits will somehow affect them negatively. For the people who fear our power, we may want to evaluate their relationship with us and explain that our choices over our eating habits does not mean that it will be harmful.

Sometimes people want to test our determination and ability to stay on a different way of eating. They will pit their cunning, guile, and deceit against our resolve and tenacity.

Just For Today: I am actively responsible for what I eat and for my improved food program. My primary responsibility is for my own growth and well-being.

We have added to our "treasure house" by changing our eating behaviors and eating to improve our health and well-being. We may have more problems with changes at one time than another, because of our body's cycles and the season of the year.

Each of us has cycles that affects how we change our lives and our weight. At least three (3) cycles influence our lives. These cycles occur **daily** (circadian rhythms), **monthly**, and **seasonally**, and occur in men as well as women.

Daily

During some hours of the day, you may be more energetic than at other times. You may consider yourself a "day person" or a "night person." You also have "hunger" levels that occur more often at one time than another. You need to discover this for yourself and learn what steps to take to avoid the trap of overeating at a time when you seem to be more hungry.

Questions to ask yourself are:

★ When do I feel most like eating more than is good for me?
★ When I wake up am I ready to eat immediately?
★ Do I feel like eating more after the sun goes down?
★ Do I want to snack all afternoon long?

From answering these questions, we find that we want to eat either more in the mornings, the afternoons, or the evenings. Snacks are scheduled to coincide more with our desires and need for additional food.

Monthly

Another cycle to know is your monthly cycle. For women, your cycle may be in relation to your menstrual cycle or other hormonal cycles. For men, your "monthly" cycle may vary from 3 weeks to 6 weeks in length. (Check this by noting and evaluating your characteristic and predominate moods each day for 3 to 6 months.)

When you know your eating cycle within your "monthly" cycle, you can readily develop strategies to overcome sabotage, relapse, or mini-binges at that time. Sometimes you "crave" sweets or chocolates, or starchy foods, or salty foods, or salty and fatty foods, or crave sweets followed by a craving for salty foods, or any combination of the above. Which of these has occurred to you? Has this caused your new eating program to be jeopardized? What strategy can you develop to overcome this urge to overdo every few weeks?

Seasonal

There are seasonal changes in our eating style, exercise habits, activities, and desires. Usually when the weather is colder we want to consume more food, and of warmer or hotter temperatures. Our body uses fat as an insulator against colder weather. This means we lose weight faster or slower on the same caloric intake because of the outside (ambient) temperatures and length of daylight. Animals insulate against cold by growing heavier, thicker coats, or adding extra fat, or both.

Knowing these cycles helps us eliminate the crazy binges, cravings, backsliding, and relapse that occur when changing and improving eating habits. When we expect "abnormal" food desires, it is much easier to develop a strategy to change and override them.

With knowledge about ourselves, we can develop the power to change our eating habits and improve our health in recovery.

SELF-POWER

In Step One, we admitted we were powerless. In Steps Two and Three we sought a Power greater than ourselves and allowed that Power to work in our lives. In Steps Six and Seven, we became ready to and asked to have our shortcomings (gluttony, anorexia, bulimia, or any other unhealthy habit) removed. We also know that our shortcomings are not removed without our conscious and consistent effort.

In eating and dieting what we thought we needed most was *will power*. What we really need is "*self-power*." Self-power or power over our actions to change is a combination of characteristics. It consists of the following:

- ★ **Know our goals.** Be very clear about our goals to change our eating habits.
- ★ **Think creatively and constructively** in situations where there is food.
- ★ **Make a decision** to achieve our goals (no half measures).
- ★ **Take suitable action** (going to any length) to achieve your goals.
- ★ **Celebrate** our successes.

> *Just For Today: I have the courage and wisdom to change and become healthier.*

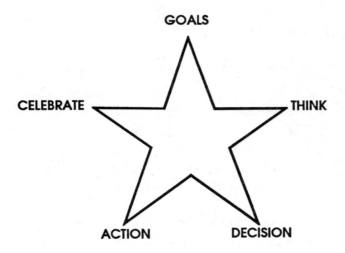

Know Our Goals

Knowing our goals and what we will do to achieve them is very important. Earlier we set not only weight goals, but health goals (cholesterol, blood pressure, etc.), appearance goals, exercise goals, and life goals. We also looked at other ambitions that sometimes interfere with achieving some of our goals. To have the "self-power" to accomplish our goals means that we are very clear about what they are.

Just For Today: I am enjoying my journey toward achievement of my weight goals and healthier eating.

Think Creatively and Constructively

We can think creatively and constructively. We easily devise a way to say "No" firmly, politely, and consistently.

Do we carry food with us for snacks? Do we eat before or after meetings? Do we have snacks out or at home? Do we plan to eat alone or with others? What are their schedules and can we fit our schedule into their plans? Keeping our routines and our lives simple helps to answer some of these questions. We can *think creatively and constructively* to keep our new lifestyle and our new program on target. When we listen, we can use intuitive guidance to progress toward healthier eating.

Perhaps in a particular situation we need to say "no." Saying "no" politely, firmly, and repeatedly is the best way to handle these people or situations. Sometimes leaving the room or situation temporarily is another way to let the matter go.

What can we say when others offer us food or are insistent that we have more or something different to eat? Some suggestions are:

"No thank you!" "Thank you, but no." Sometimes a simple statement will do the trick. "No thank you, not right now." This statement does not say NO, NEVER, but just for right now. It implies to the other person that maybe at a different time we might or would accept.

"Those do look delicious and I appreciate you offering them (one) to me, but I'll have to say no." A polite way to compliment the person who is offering us the item and a nice way to say NO.

"No thank you; I've been successful with my new eating program and want to keep my successes." This answer says no, gives you credit for the accomplishments you have made, and gives some explanation to the other person about your NO.

Now when confronted with a new or unusual eating situation we **know what to do.**

Make a Decision

We decide to implement our ideas and strategies to achieve our goals of improved health, eating better and more frequently, and exercise. We decide if we are an *action* person, a *talker*, or a *diet babbler.* We decide what physical exercises we will do and when we will do them. We decide to what lengths we will go to achieve our health goals. We decide how rapidly we will implement our strategies, where, and at what times.

In all these instances, we maintain an attitude of gratitude that we have the ability to make choices. We are polite, firm, and fair when we resolve any differences that may occur with our friends, associates, family, and peers. Whatever else we do, we decide to be consistent at each occasion and with each person. We have made a positive decision to eat healthier and exercise. *We are resolved.*

Perhaps we will share our experiences and some of our answers with others who are having the same problems we have had. Changes in our eating styles, programs, and exercise are difficult for those around us. We want to recognize their needs for affection, warmth, love, friendship, without being suffocated or engulfed in fulfilling their needs and letting ours go by the wayside. An open discussion of this topic could resolve many of the tensions and hurt feelings that may be there.

> *Just For Today: My decisions come through*
> *prayer and meditation. I readily implement*

decisions about my food, meal choices and exercise.

Take Action

Next, we take action to implement our decisions for improved health. When needed, we readily and casually say "No thank you, not now." We take action by saying "no"; by refusing to feeling uncomfortable, insecure, or frightened by the other person's reactions; and by not allowing the negative attitudes of others to have an influence over our goal.

Just For Today: I have the power to easily refuse extra food when it is offered to me.

So many times we know what we *should* do, and we have thought of a plan or way to do it, only to fail by not taking the action required at that time. We then sit back later and say to ourselves and others what we should have done. This is very much like living our lives in instant replay and correct with actions that we ought to have done but didn't.

One of the worst dreads of a person who is learning to eat differently and more healthily is that there will be a total breakdown and malfunction of their new eating program. This breakdown or malfunction starts to occur rather gradually (about 3 months into it) and seems to be of little concern initially. Then as time goes on, *it* progresses until it has snowballed into "catastrophic" and "disastrous" proportions. Total breakdowns and malfunctions happen only after certain early warning signals (symptoms analogous to relapse) have been ignored for a time. These early warning symptoms include:

★   Problems which are "not serious" or denied.

★   Continued occasions for problems which are not viewed as being serious, harmful or detrimental.

★ Failure to discuss the problem (people, places, or things) with someone else (our "cheerleader," support person, or sponsor) and to find a resolution to the situation.

★ Being arrogant and thinking that we can "take care of it ourselves" without asking for help.

> *Just For Today: I have a variety of friends that help me with my new eating approach and my healthier food choices.*

Events have a way of becoming larger and less manageable. Soon they have mushroomed into a *huge* source of pain, discouragement, worry, and potential anger. One way to put a slip into its proper perspective is to:

★ Look at the high risk situations we get into.

★ Look at where we started and where we are now.

★ Interpret what has happened.

★ Practice what we know is good for our improved health and self-esteem.

★ Evaluate our progress towards our goals.

★ Reassert our motivations and our decisions.

★ Reintroduce our creative and constructive thinking.

★ Start to take action again.

It is easy to become discouraged when we change our eating and health habits and the rest of our life does not change as rapidly. We start saying "Why bother?" A review of what we have been doing and where we are going helps to answer that question. It may also help if we look at the time of the month or year and where we would be **today** if we had not been doing anything to improve ourselves.

Over time, those of us who become discouraged but "keep on keeping on" with our new program are the ones who do very well. Those of us who give up when it is the "darkest" do not stay to see the "dawn."

> *Just For Today: I have positive expectations of reaching my health and nutrition goals, and I bounce back quickly from temporary setbacks.*

Ways to overcome these times of discouragement are to **reevaluate where we have been, what we have accomplished, where we are going, and what we will do to get there.** Decide if you are an *action* person, a *talker*, or a *diet babbler*. Review what you have learned about self-power (know your goal, think creatively and constructively, make a decision, take action, and celebrate your successes).

Celebrate

Celebrate successes! Celebrate alone or with others. Celebrating a small success helps to prevent the discouragement that may occur when you change your eating and health habits and the rest of your life does not change as rapidly. A review (inventory) of what you have been doing and where you are going helps to answer the question, "Why bother?"

Listen to what others say to you about your successes. Look at your clothes and how you fit into them differently. Determine if your slump is part of one of your body's natural cycles. Help yourself by having a friend help you. Make pleasant, positive statements to yourself. To celebrate your successes develop a list of ways to celebrate your small successes. Be creative in this area. Your ways of celebration include positive, gentle statements, activities or things to be included in your life.

> *Just For Today: I am very satisfied with my new eating program and am very pleased with my accomplishments.*

POINTS TO REMEMBER

★ We know our goals for improved health and eating.
★ We think creatively and constructively about food and eating.
★ We make decisions to achieve our goals.
★ We take action to change and achieve our goals.
★ We celebrate our successes.

EMOTIONAL REASONS WE EAT

In each day's column, check the reason(s) you are eating or want to eat. You may have more than one reason for eating at a particular time.

At the end of the week, go back and review your main reasons for eating. Is there a difference between weekends and weekdays? Now that you have an idea about your emotional reasons for eating or overeating, you can deal with those reasons and make positive changes. **Remember, food is just food.**

	WED	THU	FRI	SAT	SUN	MON	TUE
Afraid/Scared							
Angry/Mad							
Anxious/Nervous							
Bored/Restless							
Dejected/Disappointed							
Depressed/Unhappy							
Friendly/Sociable							
Frustrated							
Glad/Cheerful							
Grouchy/Irritable							
Guilty/Embarrassed							
Happy/Delighted							
Lonely/Withdrawn							
Loving/Kind							
Manipulative							
Moody/Edgy							
Nauseated/Sick							
Sad							
Uptight/Tired							
Worried/Upset							

THE TWELVE STEPS OF
ALCOHOLICS ANONYMOUS

1. We admitted we were powerless over alcohol—that our lives had become unmanageable.
2. Came to believe that a Power greater than ourselves could restore us to sanity.
3. Made a decision to turn our will and our lives over to the care of God *as we understood Him.*
4. Made a searching and fearless moral inventory of ourselves.
5. Admitted to God, to ourselves, and to another human being the exact nature of our wrongs.
6. Were entirely ready to have God remove all these defects of character.
7. Humbly asked Him to remove our shortcomings.
8. Made a list of all persons we had harmed, and became willing to make amends to them all.
9. Made direct amends to such people wherever possible, except when to do so would injure them or others.
10. Continued to take personal inventory and when we were wrong promptly admitted it.
11. Sought through prayer and meditation to improve our conscious contact with God *as we understood Him,* praying only for knowledge of His will for us and the power to carry that out.
12. Having had a spiritual awakening as the result of these Steps, we tried to carry this message to alcoholics, and to practice these principles in all our affairs.

The Twelve Steps are reprinted with permission of A.A. World Services, Inc., New York, New York.

SUGGESTED READING

Codependent No More. Melody Beattie. Harper/Hazelden. 1987.

From Chocolate to Morphine: Understanding Mind-Active Drugs. Andrew Weil, M.D., and Winifred Rosen. Houghton Mifflin Co. 1983.

Craving for Ecstasy: The Consciousness and Chemistry of Escape. Harvey Milkman and Stanley Sunderwirth. Lexington Books. 1987.

The Steps We Took. Joe McQ. August House, Inc. 1990.

A Substance Called Food. Gloria Arenson. Tab Books. 1989.

Alcoholics Anonymous (3d ed.). Alcoholics Anonymous World Services, Inc. 1976.

Recommended Dietary Allowances (10th ed.). National Academy Press. 1989.

Nutrition and Your Health: Dietary Guidelines for Americans (3d ed.). United States Department of Agriculture, United States Department of Health and Human Services. 1990.

ABOUT THE AUTHOR

Marilyn Rollins, a Registered Dietitian and Certified Diabetes Educator, has presented a number of workshops and seminars on nutrition, diet, and lifestyle changes in the recovery process. She has been a presenter for several years at the Southwestern School for Behavior Health Studies held annually in Tucson, Arizona. Marilyn is a certified instructor and has taught nutrition and weight control classes in community colleges throughout Arizona. She is practical and pragmatic when recommending and making dietary changes for a healthier life.

In addition to her many years as a nutrition/diet counselor and expert, Marilyn is a founder and owner of Gifts Anon., the oldest book and gift store for people in the 12 Step programs of recovery.

You may contact the author at:
Marilyn Rollins
c/o Gifts Anon.
4524 North Seventh Street
Phoenix, Arizona 85014-3898